INTERNATIONAL PSYCHIATRY CLINICS

SUBSCRIPTION RATE $21.50 PER YEAR. FOREIGN RATE $24.00 PER YEAR.

CLINICAL
PSYCHIATRY
AND RELIGION

EDITED BY

E. Mansell Pattison, M.D.

Department of Psychiatry
University of Washington School of Medicine, Seattle

BOSTON
LITTLE, BROWN AND COMPANY

INTERNATIONAL PSYCHIATRY CLINICS
VOL. 5, NO. 4

LIBRARY OF CONGRESS CATALOG CARD NO. 69-18016

PUBLISHED IN GREAT BRITAIN
BY J. & A. CHURCHILL LTD., LONDON

BRITISH STANDARD BOOK NO. 7000 0148 4

PRINTED IN THE UNITED STATES OF AMERICA

Contributing Authors

E. MANSELL PATTISON, M.D., Editor
Assistant Professor of Psychiatry,
Coordinator for Social and Community Psychiatry,
University of Washington School of Medicine, Seattle

CLEMENS E. BENDA, M.D.
Affiliate Professor of Abnormal Psychology,
Clark University, Worcester, Massachusetts;
Assistant Psychiatrist and Lecturer, Institute of Pastoral Care,
Department of Psychiatry, Massachusetts General Hospital, Boston

MAXWELL BOVERMAN, M.D.
Private Practice in Psychiatry, Washington, D.C.
Formerly, Clinical Professor of Psychiatry,
George Washington University, Washington, D.C.

MARGARETTA K. BOWERS, M.D.
Clinical Professor of Psychology,
Supervisor of Psychotherapy, Postdoctoral Program in
Psychotherapy, Adelphi University, Garden City, New York

ROBERT L. CASEY, M.D., Capt. U.S.M.C.
Psychiatrist, Mental Hygiene Consultation Division,
Fort Benning, Georgia

CARL W. CHRISTENSEN, M.D.
Associate, Department of Neurology and Psychiatry,
Northwestern University Medical School, Chicago;
Adjunct Professor of Pastoral Psychology,
Garrett Theological Seminary, Evanston, Illinois

RICHARD H. COX, B.D., Ph D.
Associate, Department of Neurology and Psychiatry,
Northwestern University Medical School, Chicago;
Head, Department of Psychology,
Psychologist Director, Adolescent Program,
Forest Hospital, Des Plaines, Illinois

v

EDGAR DRAPER, B.D., M.D.
Professor of Psychiatry, University of Michigan;
Director of Residency Education,
University Hospital, Ann Arbor, Michigan

TRUMAN G. ESAU, M.D.
President, Medical Staff,
Psychiatric Director, Adolescent Program,
Forest Hospital, Des Plaines, Illinois

JAMES J. GILL, M.D.
Assistant Psychiatrist, Harvard University Health Services,
Cambridge, Massachusetts;
Consulting Psychiatrist, Adolescent Unit,
Children's Hospital Medical Center, Boston

ARI KIEV, M.D.
Clinical Associate Professor of Social Psychiatry,
Head, Cornell Program in Social Psychiatry
Cornell Medical College, New York, New York

WARD A. KNIGHTS, JR., B.D., Th.D.
Teaching Chaplain, New Hampshire Hospital,
Concord, New Hampshire

ALBERT J. LUBIN, M.D.
Clinical Professor of Psychiatry,
Stanford University, Palo Alto, California

ROBERT J. MC ALLISTER, Ph.D., M.D.
Adjunct Clinical Professor,
University of Nevada, Reno;
Superintendent, Nevada State Hospital, Reno

C. F. MIDELFORT, M.D.
Lecturer in Practical Theology,
Luther Theological Seminary, St. Paul, Minnesota;
Psychiatrist, Department of Psychiatry,
La Crosse Lutheran Hospital,
La Crosse, Wisconsin

GEORGE MORA, M.D.
Clinical Associate Professor, Department of Psychiatry,
Albany Medical College, Albany, New York;
Medical Director,
The Astor Home for Children, Rhinebeck, New York

WALTER N. PAHNKE, M.D., B.D., Ph.D.
Chief of Psychiatric Research,
Maryland Psychiatric Research Center, Baltimore;
Attending Psychiatrist,
Sinai Hospital, Baltimore;
Consultant, Pastoral Counselling Centers of Greater Washington

LEON SALZMAN, M.D.
Professor of Clinical Psychiatry,
Georgetown University Medical School, Washington, D.C.;
Consultant, National Institute of Mental Health;
Lecturer, Washington School of Psychiatry, Washington, D.C.

PHILIP WOOLLCOTT, JR., M.D.
Chief of Clinical Service,
C. F. Menninger Memorial Hospital;
Consultant, Division of Religion and Psychiatry,
Menninger Foundation, Topeka, Kansas

Preface

This volume is designed to provide psychiatrists and other mental health professionals, in a variety of clinical settings, with current information on religious issues as they affect clinical practice. Although there are many theoretical discussions, as well as popular writings, there is a noticeable lack of material addressed specifically to the practicing clinician and directly to clinical issues. Our intent here is to provide information on two aspects of clinical practice: (1) what the clinician needs to know about religion in order effectively to evaluate or treat a religious patient; and (2) how the clinician can utilize religious resources and collaborate with religious personnel.

The papers are, in part, a summary of work to date. But they also ask questions, pose problems, and offer suggestions. It is my hope that the volume will stimulate further creative work on and with religion by the profession of psychiatry and our fellow mental health disciplines.

The need for data on religious issues focused on clinical concerns has been brought home to me in a variety of recent experiences. The most striking has been the experience of our psychiatric residents during training in community psychiatry. As part of their community consultation work, the residents conduct consultation to groups of ministers and to individual church programs. Among their consultation experiences, these are often the most perplexing and anxiety-producing. The residents frequently state that they have never talked with clergy before, and they wonder how they should behave; or they question how they can be of assistance in religious areas that are seen as quite foreign to psychiatric concerns; or they ask what to do about religious disagreements between themselves and the clergy, or between clergy. Many residents have little familiarity with religious concepts, institutions, or activities. Or if they have a religious affiliation, they are often little acquainted beyond their own religious tradition. Relationships between psychiatry and religion end up being interpreted within a narrow mold. Yet these consultation experiences often become the most enjoyable and rewarding in the long run. The dilemma of unfamiliarity was expressed in a departmental grand rounds presentation. Our community psychiatry residents had presented a series of consultation experiences with clergy in which they had expressed the problems of "new territory." In the subsequent discussion, several members of our department suggested that to increase psychiatric effectiveness, we might well pay attention to the teaching of religion to psychiatrists before we began teaching psychiatry to the clergy!

Other examples have come from the requests of psychiatric colleagues for information on religious problems encountered with their patients; requests from community mental health agencies for consultation on technical aspects of psychotherapy with religious patients; our departmental experience in conducting postgraduate seminars for clergymen who request not only psychiatric knowledge but assistance in specifically applying that knowledge to their unique position and problems; requests from religious communities, churches, mission boards, denominations, and so forth, for assistance in establishing psychological screening and treatment programs; and requests from religious institutions for consultation on how to apply behavioral science knowledge to religious programs —e.g., more effective small group relations, more effective education, assistance to minority groups, and social problems. In many if not all instances, the clinician is faced not with the mere transfer of psychiatric expertise, but rather with the application of clinical knowledge to the particular needs and setting within a religious framework.

The mental health community, likewise, has been casting eyes on the clergy and the church as a community mental health resource. Several mental health programs in our community, as elsewhere, have become involved in active collaboration with religious personnel and institutions in regard to both mental health problems and larger social issues. We, and others, find ourselves working on such collaboration in a very experimental fashion, for guidelines have not yet been well established, nor professional and social sanctions developed.

We have come a long way from the open suspicions, derogations, and mutual rejections that typified the earlier decades of this century. Indeed, one might feel a little uneasy over some of the too-easy rapprochement that ignores theoretical issues and clinical collaborative problems that are by no means resolved. Our intent is not to present facile solutions, but to share theoretical, experimental, and clinical explorations. I feel the other authors would concur with me that fresh understanding and creative clinical opportunities are beginning to emerge.

I hope that it will become amply evident to the reader that clinical considerations of religion have vastly expanded since the classic work of the early decades of this century. Rather than *the* psychiatric approach to religion, we have a variety of psychiatric approaches to various aspects of religion. Although I have sought to avoid becoming enmeshed in philosophical issues, not for lack of importance but for limitations of space, I have deliberately asked psychiatrists of divergent views and practices to participate in order to illustrate the variety of theoretical and clinical approaches to psychiatry and religion relationships that exist today. Further, I have sought reports by individual clinicians who have pioneered in a wide range of collaborative methods to illustrate promising avenues that lie ahead for further clinical experimentation.

As Paul Pruyser of the Menninger Clinic has recently noted, the relation between psychiatry and religion is a "polygon of relationships." It would take an entire volume to write an adequate history of the numerous skeins of clinical and theoretical work that have woven the texture of our complex scene today. Since World War II, there has been a renaissance in the scientific study of religion by psychologists, sociologists, and anthropologists that has spawned vigorous subspecialties in these professions. Likewise, the fields of pastoral psychology, pastoral counseling, and pastoral care have emerged in the same period. The richness of all these areas is beyond the scope of this volume. However, we have prepared a carefully selected bibliography, which contains pertinent books in these areas as well as more clinical references. The interested reader is referred to these for further exploration.

I am much indebted to the authors of the volume for their suggestions in addition to their own chapters. Almost all the authors have had extensive experience working with the clergy and the church; a number have had theological training. Thus they write from experience, concern, and involvement. They have reviewed and assisted in the bibliography, which represents, in a sense, a joint collaborative effort of us all. The approach to religion represented in this volume is at once subjective and objective, clinical and experimental, benevolent and skeptical, perhaps reflecting the fact that I have dealt with religious issues myself as a psychotherapist, pastor, academician, and researcher.

E. MANSELL PATTISON, M.D.

September, 1968
Seattle, Washington

Contents

xiii

CLINICAL PSYCHIATRY
AND RELIGION

PART I

CLINICAL ASPECTS OF RELIGION AND PERSONAL PSYCHOLOGY

The scientific study of religion from a psychological point of view began at the turn of the twentieth century. Academic psychologists like Ames, Coe, James, Leuba, Starbuck, and Thouless investigated the nature of mystical experiences, the psychology of conversion, and the growth of religious sentiment. Meanwhile, psychoanalytic clinicians like Freud, E. Jones, and T. Reik were studying the instinctual derivatives in religious beliefs and rituals and the ego-defensive uses of religion. In both instances only part-aspects of religion were emphasized, while the multidimensional nature of religion was overlooked. Yet the nature of religion—its taxonomy—is still to be broken down into suitable components for study. For example, C. Y. Glock and R. Stark, sociologists at Berkeley, suggest at least five "dimensions" to religion: ideological, intellectual, sacramental, experiential, and consequential. Obviously, a comprehensive psychology of religion must deal with each of these aspects.

The chapters in this section examine religion from several different viewpoints, each of which is a part-aspect. They represent various means of investigation, in part yielding complementary data, and in part demonstrating divergent emphases and conclusions.

Gill reviews experimental data on changes in religious ideation that have a maturational sequence paralleling psychosociosexual maturation. Then he addresses the issues of immature and mature religion in relation to immature and mature per-

3

sonality development. Draper uses the methods of psychoanalytic metapsychology to demonstrate that the several dimensions of religion serve a panoply of psychic functions. Further,
he shows that religion may be involved in the whole range
of intrapsychic structure and function. Benda approaches religion from an existential viewpoint, arguing that the nature
of man cannot be fully apprehended by traditional psychodynamic concepts. He suggests that existential concepts not
only enrich our understanding of religion, but also affect our
clinical view of the patient. Lubin illustrates the power of
clinical psychoanalysis in comprehending religious ideation
and behavior, carefully spelling out emendations of psychoanalytic thought and the limits of this approach. Woollcott provides a careful study of religion as it appears as part of daily
clinical psychiatry, describing how religion plays a role in
typical psychopathological processes. Pattison provides a review
of contrasting theoretical attitudes toward religion, showing
how these affect clinical practice and offering recommendations
for dealing with religion in psychotherapy. Finally, Pattison
examines the concepts of morality, guilt, and forgiveness, which
have been traditional concerns of religion; these are shown
to be integral aspects of the psychotherapeutic process.

I am sure that the theologian and the philosopher, as well
as the social scientist, would have many questions to ask of
each of these clinicians. But larger issues may require post-
ponement until we have more careful studies of the individual
psychology of religion as indicated in these chapters. The
clinical study of religion has been preoccupied with the unusual, abnormal, and defensive. These chapters extend the
clinical study of religion to the developmental, maturational,
normal, healthy, and integrative, as well.

The Psychology of Religious Development

JAMES J. GILL

BACKGROUND

By the time J. Leuba completed his *Psychological Study of Religion* (1912), he was able to quote forty-eight different definitions of religion, and to these he added several of his own. Since that time, numerous other social scientists and theologians have contributed their own variant attempts at a definition. Some, however, have concluded that religion is virtually impossible to define. The present writer feels that, for the purposes of the discussion to follow, William James (1902) provided an adequately comprehensive description by defining subjective religion as "the feelings, the acts and experiences of individual men . . . so far as they apprehend themselves to stand in relation to whatever they may consider the divine." [3]

Two discrete but related aspects of religion will be examined in this chapter. These would certainly appear deserving of consideration in the critical times and the evolving society in which we live. So much social tension, unrest, violence, crime of every sort, and widespread pessimism is evident in our nation and world today that it hardly seems surprising that many have cast a skeptical eye toward religion and demanded an accounting of its contribution or an acknowledgment of its failure to meet the urgent

5

needs of our day. The policeman on the street, the judge in his courtroom, like the conscience-searching parent in the home, wonders whether religion is able to contribute something more to the character, behavior, maturity, and stability of our people than can be credited to this agency at the present time.

Aware of widespread criticism of religious education, specialists in that field are reevaluating the manner in which religious formation has been attempted in the past. Here and abroad they have sadly watched adolescents and young adults cast aside their earlier religious beliefs and practices to think and act in a fashion that often undermines rather than confirms the values our civilization has traditionally cherished. The educators' conclusion, based on an increasing number of scientific studies of the process of religious development through childhood and adolescence, is that much of the reason for religion's failure to have a permanent and constructive effect within the personality of the individual and within society can be attributed to the fact that the presentation of religious concepts in Sunday school, in parochial school, in the synagogue, and at home has been poorly timed. Unaware of the specific limitations on the capacity for religious thinking that characterize the child at various age levels, parents and teachers have generally attempted to provide a caliber of instruction that exceeds the child's capabilities. By adolescence he often becomes both confused and bored, then expresses his dissatisfaction by rejecting religion entirely.

Research by such investigators as J. Piaget [5] and R. Goldman [1, 2], followed by the initiation of a variety of recent, innovative programs of religious instruction based on their findings, provides the basis for hope that religion may be capable of making a more significant contribution to the lives of our contemporaries and society. If so, this will be facilitated by the formulation and adoption of a more scientifically sound approach to the problem of providing a religious education for those disposed to pursue one. It would seem appropriate for psychiatrists and psychologists to become familiar with the results of these relevant developmental studies, which may contribute to potentially important changes in the thinking, feelings, and behavior of countless future adults. Consequently, the first part of this chapter will outline briefly what has been learned about the natural, age-related stages of development in religious thinking. The second part will indicate some of the ways mature religious thinking in the adult can support the maintenance of mental health in the individual and contribute to the corporate well-being of our society.

STAGES OF DEVELOPMENT IN RELIGIOUS THINKING

In considering the natural stages of development in religious thinking, there is no need to debate the question whether there is evidence compelling us to posit a special religious instinct in man. With William James and countless psychologists after him, the writer is persuaded that there is no such entity. Reflecting on religious thinking as *thinking* (which is what is intended here), I certainly do not mean to imply a denial that fantasy and feelings intimately and consistently relate themselves to this rational process. Another fact that should be noted is that the social scientist who examines religious thought within his own specialized frame of reference can rightfully say nothing about the theological truth or error of such thought as it actually occurs in the psychic life of any given individual or group. What is of concern here is the fact that religious thinking is seen to be qualitatively different at various stages of psychosociosexual development.

Mindful of the fact that religious thought (for example, about God, His actions, one's relationship with Him, the Bible, church) is stimulated in the child by the specific environment in which he lives, by his own personal experiences, and especially by the instruction and example he receives from parents and teachers, it would seem obvious that the religious thinking of each individual will be unique. Those who have extensively studied the stages of growth in religious thinking and behavior have selected children and adolescents at various age levels, all of whom had some exposure to the religious thinking of others, generally communicated in the form of Bible-centered instruction in church, at school, or at home. Obviously, the more nearly homogeneous the subjects' environments and the type and extent of their religious indoctrinations, the more accurate and meaningful could be the conclusions drawn by investigators.

One of the outstanding contributions of J. Piaget has been the schematic representation he has provided with regard to the developmental stages of the thinking process in general. He has demonstrated that children and adolescents, although varying somewhat from individual to individual, organize and interpret their experiences according to a relatively constant motivational pattern. He has called the first two years of life "the period of sensori-motor intelligence." Despite the fact that language and memory appear in this phase, no evidence of religious thinking is presented. It is not until the "intuitive phase," extending from years 2 to 7, that Piaget notes the first stage of thought that is specifically religious. He points out, however, that two factors severely limit the child's understanding of religious matters. The first is his *egocentricity*, his tendency to interpret all reality exclusively in terms of what happens immediately to himself. The second restricting factor is his *concretization*, or the inclination to concentrate his thinking on physical and materialistic data, with relative inability to think abstractly, understand metaphors, or deal with hypotheses. With regard to the child's earliest religious-like activities, such imitative behavior as bowing the head or folding the hands in a prayerful posture is actually no more consciously religious than such actions as drinking from a cup or waving good-bye to someone.

Piaget describes the period extending from ages 4 to 7 as one of "mythological artificialism." Celestial bodies, clouds, storms, and rivers are thought to originate by divine, if not human, agency. The sun, for example, may be seen as a fire lit by God using a match. It is at about age 5 that the child begins to accept the power of God as explanation for all things. God is thought to be omnipotent and in complete control of all natural forces.

Among the investigations of the developmental stages in religious thinking, some of the most extensive and perhaps the most interesting work has been accomplished by R. Goldman [1, 2]. Using pictures, Scripture stories, and interviews, he studied several hundred children and adolescents, ages 6 through 17, dividing them into four stages of development according to his results. His observations, in general, confirm those of other researchers, including J. Piaget, E. Harms, R. Loomba, and M. Argyle. I will attempt to summarize very briefly in the next several paragraphs the general nature of their findings.

Early Childhood (ages 5 to 7)

God is construed by children at this stage as an omnipotent, fatherly figure, infallible and able to be trusted completely. His powers are thought to be like those of a magician. Fantasy helps to produce such charming statements as the one Goldman records: "God is in the sky and you can't see him. He flies around. Sometimes he stops behind a cloud to have something to eat. He goes down to land at night to see shepherds and to talk to them." The child has a natural sense of the numinous, or mysterious and awesome nature of God. At this age his prayers are generally simple requests for material favors, but his feeling about prayer is usually quite strong. The Bible, if encountered during this stage, is given special respect and treated almost as if the book possessed some magical quality. It is accepted as written personally by God or *one* powerful, holy person, and is therefore regarded as literally and entirely true.

Middle Childhood (ages 8 to 9)

Even though inductive and deductive thinking have generally begun by about age 7, thought is still limited principally to "concrete" situations, actions, and sensory data. Piaget places the thinking of children at this stage within the type he calls "technical artificialism," in which a natural explanation is joined with an artificial solution. An example of such thinking would be that provided by a child in Goldman's study who considered the moon to be a condensation of clouds, but the clouds had been made by

God. Children at this stage will not debate whatever religious explanation a parent or teacher presents to them; agnosticism is unthinkable at this age. Goldman found that God is typically thought of as a man of large stature, attired in long, flowing robes, with a powerful voice, living in the sky and making sorties to earth. His visits are not thought to occur as frequently now as they did in Bible times. God is seen as sometimes angry and vindictive, as well as unpredictable. Only at times is He kind and loving. God is also constantly frighteningly just, and His edicts are issued principally in the form of prohibitions. Childish fantasy and animistic thinking (that natural objects are *alive*) are fading during this stage, while the elements of reality are increasingly compelling acceptance. However, literal belief in angels continues, these being conceived as real people with physical substance and palpable wings. The Bible is considered as a holy book, either written by God or authorized by Him, and true in every detail because of its divine authorship. Scriptures are interpreted in a primitive, literal, and concretistic way. The child perceives no distinction between what is written in the Bible as history and what is myth, legend, allegory, or poetry. God and Jesus are often confused in the minds of children, their names being used interchangeably. Jesus is frequently addressed in prayers, but he is not appreciated as a real man. Prayer is generally found pleasurable and reflects materialistic desires and a residual egocentricity. Regarding religious and moral behavior at this stage, the child accepts adults' decisions about what is right or wrong, with the authority of parents yielding gradually to that of teachers. The child has no real insight into the nature of evil. Being *bad* is simply acting contrary to a rule or command.

Late Childhood and Preadolescence (ages 9 to 12)

During this period, as experience with life increases, many children go through episodes of considerable intellectual confusion as they attempt to formulate a more realistic and less fantastic theology. God is seen now as supernatural rather than just superhuman. A very real problem of this age group is that of God's being *everywhere* and yet at one place at one particular time. Many children, beginning at about age 10, develop a dualistic view of life, especially of the natural world. What pertains to the divine is conceived as related to the realm of magic and the long ago; modern living is recognized as hinged to the laws of nature, and God is nowhere to be seen. The child does not suspect an opposition between these two worlds, but neither does he detect a relationship between them. While God's action in the world is still being thought of as predominantly occurring in the past, the Bible continues to be an authority to be interpreted in the literal, verbal sense. However, the fact of its multiple authorship can now be accepted.

The deity is pictured as far off "in heaven," but now as a Being endowed with power and glory, rather than concretely as a man. He is still more concerned with vengeance than with love. Yet, by the end of this period, many children are close to realizing that divine love and justice are actually compatible. Earlier in childhood, "the devil" was, like God and angels, envisioned anthropomorphically. Now he is conceptualized as the diabolical spirit who is able to motivate wicked men to perpetrate monstrously evil deeds. Jesus is seen as a supermagician until about age 13. There is very little understanding of his mission or the contemporary relevance of his message. Regarding morality, Goldman [2] points out: "the Golden Rule of 'Do unto others as you wish them to do to you' needs no overt religious sanction behind it, for it is evident common sense to pupils at this stage of their social development."

Adolescence (age 13 upward)

With the child now capable of thinking in more abstract terms ("formal operational thinking," as Piaget calls it), development in this stage is characterized by the jettisoning of childish modes of thought and the development of a more adult range of interests, curiosity, and style of thinking. Their greatly increased intellectual ability now allows adolescents to advance toward solid and mature thought and behavior in the religious aspect of their lives, just as in the social, sexual, and academic spheres. This progress is reflected in their more adult concepts of God, Jesus, evil, prayer, and the church. Goldman has found that the potential for religious growth is actualized more often by the adolescents who are intellectually brighter, and, interestingly, more often by girls than by boys.

The Bible is now comprehended less literally, and God is understood in abstract and symbolic terms. Recognized as spirit, He is thought of as unseen and unseeable. His communications are appreciated as internal to the recipient, not requiring that God employ a human voice. At this stage, with the adolescent finally in possession of a developed sense of time, the historical continuity manifested in the Bible is able to be comprehended.

Everyone familiar with adolescents knows that peer values are of enormous importance to them, and the authority of adults is challenged by them almost relentlessly. Nevertheless, the teen-age boy or girl is in search of a moral authority, and often a gnawing tension exists between the need for certainty and the need to be, at the same time, independent. It has been pointed out by a number of behavioral scientists that adolescence is more a period of decision than of increased religious activity. It is during this period that young people decide whether to accept or reject their membership in the church of their parents. Statistics from recent years reveal that increasing numbers have chosen to reject affiliation rather than maintain it. As mentioned earlier, many authorities in the field of religious education now feel that this act of abandonment of membership and belief is all too often the end product of excessively zealous attempts to introduce children to religious concepts which are beyond their capacity to integrate into their thinking at their current age.

RELIGIOUS MATURITY

Just as in childhood and adolescence religious thinking and behavior (for example, prayers, churchgoing, hymns, art, drama) contribute to the satisfaction of such basic needs as security, fantasy, community, meaning, idealism, and love, in adulthood, too, religion can and obviously does make comparable contributions. If the normal stages of psychosociosexual maturation have been negotiated successfully, the individual is in possession of the personality endowment prerequisite for religious maturity. There are undoubtedly some otherwise quite mature adults whose religious thinking, because of limited instruction or interest, has remained immature, and perhaps even childish. But true religious maturity is inconceivable apart from emotional maturity in general. Moreover, stable and profound religious thought and sentiment can add dimension and richness to the quality of one's maturity. It has been the writer's experience as a physician to encounter a large number of deeply religious persons of various "faiths" whose mental health appeared to be strongly supported by the elements comprising their personal religious beliefs and practices. On the other hand, experience with neurotic and psychotic individuals, as well as with many suffering from the various types of character disorders, has provided striking evidence of the lack of such supporting elements in their lives. These are excessively anxious, pessimistic, withdrawn, or hostile adults who had either failed to develop the religious aspect of their psychic life or had for some reason abandoned it along the way.

Needs and Attitudes

It would seem appropriate in this final section to mention a few of these religious elements that appear to contribute significantly to emotional maturity or stability in mental health. Perhaps the most potent adjunct to emotional strength and equanimity, amid the inevitably stressful vicissitudes of contemporary existence, is the conviction that there exists a paternal deity, omniscient and omnipotent, with whom the individual is able to communicate (for example, through prayer or sacrament) and by whom he feels he is personally known and loved. The need to feel known and the need to feel loved are as relentlessly demanding as they are real within the deepest psychic core of every mature adult. These are paralleled by an equally essential need to find others lovable as well as responsive. On the same deep level of the mature personality, there is the need to perceive that one's own life is somehow meaningful and important in the context of an intelligible and integrated universe. The developed mind, beginning in adolescence, hungers for a sense of the significance of life's events taken collectively as well as in their singularity. Some vast *totality* that will somehow help to explain the death of a loved one just as readily as it does the changes in the seasons or the color of the sky is the object of every mature mind's spontaneous search for an integrated philosophy of existence. The minds of men keep grasping for truth while their hearts go on craving for love. The fulfillment of these needs and the activation of these potentialities is facilitated for many by the agencies of religious thinking and behavior; so is the continuing pursuit of self-development in virtue, or "character."

It is *healthy,* any student or therapist of human nature must surely agree, for a man to view the world around him as an incomplete creation, open to further imaginative, productive, rewarding activity on his part. Such an outlook is fostered in many by their religious beliefs. As a result, they live their lives with constancy and enthusiasm, with society deriving benefits from their optimism and industry. Furthermore, the individual whose faith assures him that he has precious worth and is loved by his all-powerful, concerned God can relax with a sense of trust—a feeling that his own efforts at living a good and productive life are being supported by a provident, protecting, and well-pleased Father. Such a man, experience shows us, is generally relatively free from the feelings of worthlessness and guilt that characterize clinical depression. Not that a deeply religious person cannot become depressed, or anxious, or withdrawn, of course. Rather, the man whose self-esteem is reinforced by the conviction that he is approved and loved by God and that his worth is unquestionable, no matter how limited his success, fame, or possession of material goods, is defended against the tendency to feel insignificant and a failure—even in a world where he lives buried, as hundreds of millions of us do, in the mass society of today, where worth tends to be confused with wealth and the common man must struggle to stave off feelings of political and social impotence.

For another way in which religion can be of service to psychic maturity, there is evidence that the believer who has grown to regard his God as forgiving finds it more readily possible to demand less than perfection from himself and to forgive the flaws in his own behavior. The conviction that God can still love him despite his imperfect performance serves as a defense against relentless and insatiable superego demands. The expectation that special assistance from *above* will be available in times of unusual distress or need provides yet another defense against excessive anxiety about the future. Moreover, those who cherish the belief that their lives, despite apparent death, will in some way (related to the *soul*) go on forever, and that a heaven of unalloyed happiness awaits them, are in a position to become and remain less anxiously concerned about milking pleasure from every hour of earthly existence. They are better defended against experiencing the unprofitable, sibling-rivalry type of pain that results from envying others who are more prosperous. In general, such religious persons are more readily able to accept their lot in this brief life "here below."

Those who believe that physical and emotional suffering can be, in some mysterious way, salutary and even meritorious are probably better endowed than anyone else to survive the psychic stress of debilitating injury or chronic illness without developing severe depression. Again, those whose religion provides them with certitude that their God can strengthen the sufferer, mitigate his pain, or even heal him miraculously would seem better equipped than many to cope with incurable illness or any temporary distress that is severe. If they are truly confident that God is able to hear and is inclined to reply to their urgent prayers, they can potentially experience *hope* on a level unattainable by the unbeliever. Moreover, if their beliefs also include the existence of such protecting figures as saints and angelic spirits, loneliness is a little less likely to overwhelm them. Similarly, prayer directed toward those who have already "passed into the next life" can serve to decrease one's fear of the experience of death, as well as one's anxiety about going into oblivion.

Social Functioning

When religious enlightenment assists a person to maintain consistent, realistic self-esteem based upon appreciation of himself as unique and destined to enjoy an eternal beatitude, the development of a profound regard for others as possessing comparable value and significance is facilitated. Social functioning is encouraged by this positive sort of attitude toward one's fellowmen, and withdrawal into hostile isolation becomes less likely. Sincere concern for the life-needs of others, together with generous dedication to the alleviation of their varied forms of distress—characteristic religion-fostered attitudes—will tend to motivate activities that will both solidify interpersonal relationships and gratify one's *need to be needed.* This mature, practical, unselfish love of one's neighbor can serve powerfully to counterbalance the inner forces of potentially destructive aggression that might otherwise generate agonizing violence within the individual as well as in society.

Just as aggressive impulses are often channeled by religious persons into socially acceptable and constructive enterprises, their sexual drive, too, is often given expression by them in sublimated form. Numerous traditional cultic observances of organized religion give evidence of this underlying dynamic. Moreover, the value religious persons place upon life itself is often reflected in their corresponding attitude toward sexuality. Many look upon reproduction, a creative activity, as affiliating the participants with the creator-diety. The same sexual behavior that is open to exploitation or even brutality becomes for many an occasion for the elevation of their sense of freedom and responsibility to its highest point in their lives. Also, the experience of parenthood provides opportunities and obligations religious individuals frequently regard as sacred and pertaining to the noblest level of emotionality. One's religious motivation to be a genuinely helpful and faithful spouse as well as an exemplary parent can promote responsible rather than impulsive behavior, thus tending to stabilize one's marriage and society, while at the same time reinforcing the quality of one's emotional maturity.

Psychological Support

In addition to influencing a believer and society in such potentially beneficial ways as those mentioned above, religion at times lends itself to an individual's pathological requirements and manifests itself in his psychiatric symptomatology. These diverse uses of the elements of religion have been given consideration in a recent publication by the Group for the Advancement of Psychiatry [6]. Today the imperiled emotional well-being of adults, adolescents, and children, as well as society itself, in a period of severe civil, racial, economic, and international turbulence suggests a continued and intensified study of the psychological aspects of religion and an application of the findings of this research to the task of promoting emotional development and mental health. Such a clinical attitude toward religion prescinds, of course, from its primary aim—the fostering of a relationship with the deity. Still, an appreciation of religion as a potential preventive and therapeutic adjunct may at times prove extremely useful to the clinician. Whether or not the practicing psychiatrist of today can statistically confirm from his own clinical observations the following statement of C. G. Jung [4], it still remains one that perhaps deserves serious consideration:

Among all my patients in the second half of life—that is to say, over thirty-five—there has not been one whose problem in the last resort was not that of finding a religious outlook on life. It is safe to say that every one of them fell ill because he had lost that which the living religions of every age have given to their followers, and none of them has been really healed who did not regain his religious outlook.

REFERENCES

1. Goldman, R. *Religious Thinking from Childhood to Adolescence.* London: Routledge, & Kegan Paul, 1964.
2. Goldman, R. *Readiness for Religion.* New York: Seabury, 1968.
3. James, W. *Varieties of Religious Experience.* London: Longmans, Green, 1928.
4. Jung, C. G. *Modern Man in Search of a Soul.* London: Kegan Paul, 1936.
5. Piaget, J. *The Child's Conception of the World.* London: Routledge, & Kegan Paul, 1929.
6. The psychic function of religion in mental illness and health. *Group Advance. Psychiat.* [*Rep.*] 67, 1968.

Psychological Dynamics of Religion*

EDGAR DRAPER

INTRODUCTION

A current challenge for the scientific psychological investigation of religion is to bring to bear on the study of religion those psychological studies of Freud and other investigators that unlatched doors of investigation, which still remain ajar but not yet fully open. This paper is admittedly a one-sided examination that attempts to scrutinize religion as it is experienced as an intrapsychic and completely individualized affair. Looking at religion as it is experienced intrapsychically is facilitated by the systematic methodological application of the several metapsychological points of view.

Metapsychology's value to the surveillance of religion should be no different from its scrutiny of or attempt to explain *any* mental act or function. Thus, any mentation—conscious, unconscious, spiritual, aesthetic, moral, inspiring, or emotional—theoretically has a base of understanding in an intrapsychic framework. Put in other words, each person's mind *does something with* and responds to the outside world's stimuli, including religious ones. Further discussion of the theoretical justifications and cautions for the use of metapsychological methods is beyond the scope of this paper. This has been elaborated in the author's related papers [5, 6, 7] and in the

* An expanded version of this paper will be published in the *Cincinnati Journal of Medicine*. This abbreviated version is published with their permission.

discussions of Brierley [2], Rapaport and Gill [30], Waelder [32], and Kohut [25]. With no claim to comprehensiveness, I wish, rather, to illustrate a metapsychological approach to religious data as it is brought into the foci of the several systems of the mind, including the topographical, dynamic, economic, genetic, structural, and adaptive points of view.

THE TOPOGRAPHICAL POINT OF VIEW

Inherent in Freud's topographical model as outlined in the classic seventh chapter of "The Interpretation of Dreams" [9] are not only concepts of the realms of unconscious, preconscious, and conscious thinking; there also are elucidations of primary and secondary processes and the place of the primitive mental mechanisms (symbolization, condensation, displacement, and transference). From studies of infants and children and from observations of psychotic patients, the primitive processes of condensation, transference, displacement, and symbolization appear to antedate the period called by Hartmann [22] "object differention." When one considers psychological functioning in its normal developmental evolution, these primary process expressions inferentially begin before the ego is well differentiated and persist as a normal operation after differentiation, e.g., in transference phenomena.

In consideration of mental functioning, to think of transference in the grossly restricted sense of the therapeutic situation, or even as expanded to include the transfer of old psychological cathexis from a parent to a present person not in the therapeutic situation, is to see only the top of the transference iceberg. As Kohut [25] has so clearly reminded us, "Freud's basic definition of transference is: the influence of the unconscious upon the preconscious across an existing (though often weakened) repression barrier. Dreams, symptoms and aspects of the perception of the analyst by the analysand are the most important forms in which transference appears" (to the analyst!). Transference is the move from an unconscious memory or idea on to an idea in the preconscious, forming there what

Kohut has called "an amalgam." Freud [9] added that a repressed (unconscious) idea resembled that of an American dentist in his own country who could only practice under the license (cover) of an M.D., a stalking horse, who gave the dentist a ride. He adds that dream residues not only borrow something from the unconscious (the instinctual force of the repressed wish), *they offer something in return,* that is, the necessary *point of attachment for a transference.* Freud makes it clear that the phenomenon of transference is a normal mentation process [9]. It does not wait for nor need an analyst to come along. It operates in dream formation. I would add in religious formations, too. Thus, a patient's transference may be made to a theological concept, a belief, a dogma, a priest, a saint, a ritual, a prayer, a set of beads, an ethic, an order, a tradition, a sacrament, a fellowship, a hymn, a Bible verse, story, or character, a disciple or charismatic person, like Jesus, Buddha, or Muhammed.

I was struck in an earlier study [7] of 50 randomly chosen psychiatric patients, most of whom were not hospitalized, by the opulence of their ideational investment and affective attachment to some aspect or other of religion. Yet they were not in the least qualified by us or themselves as suffering from "religiosity." With a few exceptions, they could not be considered even religious in any seriously committed way. Ostow [29] has reported similar observations regarding a number of analytic cases who were not only areligious but "atheistic," yet demonstrated certain cathexes in a religious form of one kind or another as expressions of drive-derivative satisfactions. He concluded that absence of a formal religious identification was no bar in the least to what he summed up as "a need to believe." Our own study [7] made it clear that religion, with its great variety of forms, can serve as an external attachment for psychological conflict; for clinical revelation of the varieties of psychosexual developmental attainment; for ego, superego, and id operations; for grossly primitive magical pregenital and perhaps preobject expressions; as well as for highly sophisticated secondary process activity, reflected in the formulations of the most psychosexually well-developed of theologians.

Further, there appears to be a distinct similarity in the function of psychological phenomena that occurs with individual cathexes in art, fraternal or secret orders, political parties, totems, fetishes, transitional objects, and the day residue of dreams. All these offer external "innocent" opportunity for internal psychological cathexes. Each person's cathexis in any one of these stalking horses, though there may be "orthodoxy" on the surface, is completely personalized, unique, and individually determined. Each of these external "carriers" serves as a point of attachment for either unconscious or preconscious mentation.

Ernst Kris has observed in his paper "On Preconscious Mental Processes" [27]: "the absolution from guilt for fantasy is complete if the fantasy is not one's own. This accounts for the role of the bard in primitive society, and in part for the function of fiction, drama, etc., in our society." Included in his "etc." has to be religion. The service of these cultural inheritances "is guiltlessly borrowed" by individuals for discharge, regression, and catharsis.

Freud [10], in commenting on a decisive step in dream formation, said, "The preconscious dream wish is formed, which gives expression to the unconscious impulse in the material of the preconscious day's residues." Thus the dream wish is not the same as the impulse, though it is expressive of it, but finds its manifestation closest to the surface in the day residue. This is part of the "dream work." Freud also found similar work being done in humor and by jokes, or "joke work." A veritable stable of stalking horses available in religions makes "religious work" a mental operation easily understood through topographical perspectives.

THE PSYCHODYNAMIC POINT OF VIEW

Rapaport and Gill [30] define this point of view as an interplay of psychological forces that may work together or at odds (conflict) with each other, but the final effect is determined by the outcome of the direction and magnitude of each.

Freud's major works about religion must be considered too generalized a treatment of the subject to qualify as scientific. He looked for broad principles that would be applicable to the masses. Although we would concede that the Oedipus complex, for example, may play a role in a certain individual's religious position, or his ideas of God, it is, as shown in our previous study, not the *only* and perhaps not even the *central* developmental conflict that is played out in the religious realm. It is in the data of the case that we can be definitive about the interplay of internal psychological forces that make dynamics come alive.

It would be erroneous to be hoodwinked into thinking Freud did not, in works other than these general ones, focus on psychodynamic aspects of religion as studied in individual cases. In his article "A Religious Experience" [11], he analyzed the conversion experience of an American doctor as reported to him by letter. In his careful study of the "Wolfman" [12], he took pains to translate the meaning of religion for his patient as a little boy. He linked concepts of ambivalence and obsessive acts dynamically with the religious acts of kissing holy pictures, the making of the cross, and repetition of "God-shit" thoughts. The sadomasochism of the passion story, hating God, getting the Holy Ghost, and the Wolfman's identification with Christ as submissive to the will of God the Father, all became understood in the revealing light of psychoanalytic dynamics.

Freud understood Schreber's religious preoccupations to reflect "a method in his madness." In a man who had been no believer in a personal God before he became ill, Schreber's voluptuous affair with and marriage to the God of the "anterior and posterior realms" who could offer "male and female states of bliss" found earthbound explanations in Freud's enlightened perceptions [13].

In our earlier study [7], it became clear that the vicissitudes of life altered the choice of an individual's religious interests; that is, what is important one year in one's religion may not be important in the next year. The current life situation, age, and stage of the individual offer precipitating possibilities for unwitting choice within the wide provisions of religious doctrines, rituals, and so forth. For instance, in a patient known to be suffering with chronic thanatophobia, fears of "going to hell" arose when he neared completion of an important project or a success. These fears were fed by castration anxiety, secondary to his oedipal rivalry with his father. Fears of *extinction* loomed, however, when possibilities occurred of interruption of a current sadomasochistic relationship, which had its origin in his genetically earlier separation fears stemming from his near-symbiotic relationship with his mother.

Our study made it clear that in order to understand the psychological place religion plays for any one person, we must take into account his psychosexual development, character structure, current conflicts, and whatever his exposures have been to the great variety of experiences with a religious coloring in his life. Although Freud was addressing himself to creative thinking and daydreaming, this principle of dynamic understanding, that is, current precipitants, is affirmed. "We must not suppose that the products of this imaginative activity—various phantasies, castles in the air and daydreams —are stereotyped or unalterable. On the contrary, they fit themselves into the subject's shifting impressions of life, with every change in his situation, and receive from every fresh active impression what might be called a 'date-mark' "[13]. One's personal philosophy or religious interests are equally molded by life's experiences.

THE ECONOMIC POINT OF VIEW

The psychoanalytic explanation of phenomena that deals with psychological energy is called the economic point of view. As Rapaport and Gill have outlined it, it assumes finite quantitative measurements, however imprecise, of energies that enter psychological operations; these energies follow laws of conservation and entropy and are subject to transformation as in processes of neutralization, sublimation, sexualization, and aggressivization [30].

Freud sheds much light on our understanding of this economic point of view. Speaking of a case that "would not have been classified as persecutory paranoia, apart from analysis," Freud's observations taught him that classical persecutory ideas may be present without great investment, but "flash up occasionally during the analysis." He adds, "It seems to me that we have here an important discovery—namely, that the qualitative factor, the presence of certain neurotic formations, has less practical significance than the quantitative factor, the degree of attention, or, more correctly, the amount of cathexis that these structures are able to attract to themselves. . . . Thus, as our knowledge grows, we're increasingly impelled to bring the *economic* point of view into the foreground" [15]. Continuing this discussion of paranoia in a later paper, he adds, "The cure of such paranoic attacks would lie not so much in a resolution and correction of the delusional ideas as in a withdrawal from them of the cathexis which has been lent to them." Such shifts of cathexis "would have to be brought in to explain a whole number of phenomena belonging to normal mental life." Freud cautiously extends such a principle to explanations of humor [16]. I would add the treasure house of religion as a rich resource in which such cathectic shifts can be observed. Would this principle, for example, not apply to those patients who suffer with chronic or intermittent religiosity (hyperinvestment in religious forms)? Recognizing what is behind such shifts, we cannot then hold Mary, Jesus, Buddha, or God (dead or alive) responsible, any more than we could Napoleon, as the *source* of delusions or psychopathology.

A dramatic place, too, in addition to the phenomena of religiosity and religious delusions, to witness the economic aspects of religious operations is in conversion episodes. Christensen's [4] careful clinical study concludes that the conversion experience is a "special instance of the acute confusional state" as described by Helen Carlson [3]. The ego is overwhelmed either transiently or more permanently in such episodes. Whether transient or more permanent confusion results depends not on the immediate energetic explosiveness of the experience but on its management by the individual ego. This depends upon the health of the ego prior to such experiences and, more particularly, on its capacity for draining and filtering energetic charges through neutralization, as described so well by Hartmann [21].

Kurt Eissler [8], after acknowledging his own skepticism of mir-

acles, adds, "But I am convinced that the Savior cured schizophrenia in the acute phase." (The cure of the second stage, or "mute
stage," of schizophrenia, which he notes to be omitted from the
Gospels, is another, more pessimistic story.) Eissler thought the
effectiveness of the therapist's impact on the acute schizophrenic
was directly proportional to the charismatic similarity of the therapist to Jesus. Without all of his tongue in his cheek, he adds, "I
only wonder why the churches which usually guard their preroga-
tives with jealousy, so easily surrendered to science the privilege of
treating schizophrenics."

Getting the attention of the acutely disturbed, energetically
flooded patient appears to be made easier by the conveyance of the
therapist's omnipotence, "real" (as felt by the therapist) or fantasied. My first exposure to the Black Muslims came in 1954, at
Cincinnati General Hospital, when a powerfully built, maniacally
homicidal, Negro patient was forced into a seclusion room by four
huge but badly bruised orderlies and guards. Much to the orderlies'
consternation, I said that I wanted to go in and talk to the patient.
They wondered who was crazier. To make a long story short, I was
not nearly charismatic enough to quiet him. But just a few minutes
later the patient's pastor arrived and introduced himself to me as
"Mr. X." I asked him, in my ignorance, "How do you spell that—
E-C-K-S?" And his *charisma* shone. He announced his intent to talk
with the patient and, reluctantly, we all went in again. But this
time, on sight of his leader, the patient's psychotic fury disappeared
as fast as a bursting bubble, and he docilely yielded to his pastor's
command, "Put up with the white man for now." If there ever was
a "double whammy" applied, this was it. For the remainder of this
now icily cold, rage-torn, but superficially cooperative schizophrenic
patient's hospitalization, Mr. X was a much-welcomed visitor.

The processes of libidinal sublimation, contained in religious
expressions, can be seen in limpid-eyed teen-age girls in youth
groups singing the hymn, "I walk in the Garden alone, while the
dew is still on the roses, and the voice I hear falling on my ear, to
me the Son of God discloses, and He walks with me and He talks
with me, and He tells me I am His own, and the joy we share as

we tarry there, none other has ever known." There is no shortage of sublimated aggression, either, in observing the militaristic pleasure of latency-aged boys marching around a Sunday school class with guns on shoulders, singing, "Onward Christian soldiers, marching as to war."

THE GENETIC POINT OF VIEW

Rapaport and Gill define the genetic point of view as the pscho-analytic explanation of phenomena that includes propositions concerning the psychological origins and developments of those phenomena. Such explanations describe why a specific solution was adopted, what its psychosexual developmental contribution is, and what pathways of maturation have been followed through use of innate givens, such as autonomous ego functions [30]. Clearly, they do not limit their genetic point of view to psychosexual development of Freud's "Three Essays" alone, but broaden it to include Hartmann's concepts of ego psychology and its autonomous functioning. Although these concepts belong together, our focus here will dwell upon developmental aspects, saving Hartmann's elaborations for the structural and adaptational models.

The two pillars of Freud's attention to religion seem to be the Oedipus complex and "religion of Western people," as defined in "The Future of an Illusion" [17]. This summation, "which roughly corresponds to the final form taken by our present-day white Christian civilization," turns out to be a particular brand of pietistic Protestantism not now in great prominence. I do not believe these two pillars (that is, his constricted view of Western religion and the Oedipus complex) are nearly enough to support the great cathedral of religious psychology. It must be supported additionally by the whole console of psychosexual stages of development. (Further, it must include the spectacular breadth of religion in its myriad forms of sects, cults, varieties of faiths, and infinite possibilities of cathexis within even any one denominational position.)

Our previous study [7] of 50 randomly chosen patients included the gamut of developmental types from the most infantile to definite oedipal ones, as well as formal religious identifications that ranged from belligerent atheists, through indifferent agnostics, to varieties of Catholic, Protestant, Jewish, and Buddhist identifications.

I would like to cite a brief excerpt from the summary of a case from that study that reflected no signs of having made any developmental excursion as far advanced up the scale as Oedipus:

CASE 5. This 19-year-old Pentecostal woman attended "church picnics every week." She stated that her mother felt strongly that "by faith we will be healed," and that her mother had seen others healed at religious meetings. Her favorite Bible story was "Exodus —when Jesus (sic) came and took all the people away from Egypt and led them out to the land of milk and honey." Her favorite Bible character was "Jesus—who miraculously fed the multitudes." She felt God's function was to answer prayers of request. She found that faith and communion ("you know, the bread and the grape juice") meant the most to her in her religion. She looked forward to going to heaven, which is "not the same as here." Her favorite Bible verse was, "I will lift up my eyes unto the Lord, my help cometh from the Lord." The powerful wishes to be fed and cared for, and the orientation around mother and God as givers of food and support, were viewed as a consolation fantasy resulting from unfulfilled dependency wishes. The lack of conflict over the wishes to be taken care of, together with the depressed, fatalistic outlook, the helplessness, and the use of religion for nourishment and magical thinking pointed toward a fixed oral dependent character without an inkling of a developmental excursion into Oedipus.

One of the clear upshots of our study can be summarized as follows: Individuals with psychosexual development of a primitive nature adopt equally primitive religious cathexes, which can be sufficiently revealing to allow one to make genetic diagnoses from their religious data alone.

THE STRUCTURAL POINT OF VIEW

Rapaport and Gill indicate that the psychoanalytic explanation of the structural point of view includes propositions concerning the abiding configurations (structures) involved in a psychological phenomenon. These structures (ego, id, and superego, or "mental apparatus" of Hartmann) change slowly and interact together, differentiate developmentally but with autonomous possibilities [30].

The persistent focus of the literature on the psychopathological, dynamic, and superego aspects of religion is a surprising phenomenon not unlike the "cultural lags" that Arlow and Brenner [1] have noted regarding certain other aspects of the psychoanalytic theory involving the structural model. Perhaps this lag may be due in part to the inertia of psychoanalytic investigations to move from Freud's two pillar positions (a delimited view of religion and the Oedipus complex) and to those tendencies of his to view religion in all its ramifications as pathological. Some psychiatrists still find religion worthy only of eradication in their patients and pursue its excision as vigorously as a preacher might pursue sin, or a surgeon cancer. (Naturally, however, when a psychological conflict gets itself hitched to religious expressions, that is a different story.) On the other side of the coin, we know of therapists who do not wish to tamper with the "sacred" and thus allow the defensive possibilities of religious investment to remain untouched. Religion is still by no means a neutral phenomenon of psychological interest, as seems to be more the case with a patient's artistic cathexes.

In "The Ego and the Id" [19], Freud asserts, "As a substitute for a longing for the father, the superego contains the germ from which all religions have evolved. Religion, morality, and a social sense— chief elements in the higher side of man—were originally one and the same thing." In "Totem and Taboo," [18] he had traced these back phylogenetically to the father of the primal horde. But he goes on to say, "The question is: what was it, the ego of primitive man or his id, that required religion and morality in those early days out of the father complex? Or are we wrong in carrying the differentiation between the ego, superego and the id back into such early times? Or should we not honestly confess that our whole conception of the processes in the ego is of no help in understanding phylogenesis and cannot be applied to it?" [19] It is not hard to understand in the light of Freud's two pillar foci how he could declare

Immanuel Kant's "categorical imperative" to be "the direct heir of the Oedipus complex." But does such a condensation really account for that magnificent philosopher's ego-integrative capacities, which are required for such elaborate productions as his? Freud's interest in understanding phylogenesis need not stand in the way of our understanding religion's relationship to the ego, the id, and the superego, as Hartmann [21] suggests.

Both in our earlier study and in this one we have harped on the principle of individualization. Freud had stated [15] that religious ideas in the widest sense are "perhaps the most important item in the psychical inventory of a culture." Our previous study indicated that although formal religions must reflect a culture, they certainly do not necessarily reflect the individual [7]. Hartmann and Lowenstein, in their "Notes on the Superego" [24], add their authority to this principle of individualization as it concerns the structural point of view. They note that the value hierarchy is authentic not because value systems are in the culture, but because they are consonant with the "individual psychological background"; and further, "despite the influence of sociocultural factors there remains the fact that the personal moral codes testify to the characteristics of the personality who holds them in the same way as his instincts and his ego do."

THE ADAPTIVE POINT OF VIEW

The adaptive point of view, as outlined by Rapaport and Gill [30], includes those propositions that concern relationships to the environment. There is the assumption that every point in the life cycle of an individual calls for psychological states of adaptation that insure survival and mesh with that individual's particular society, and that there are mutually influential exchanges between the society and that individual.

Religion may serve as stalking horse not only for intrapsychic projections, but equally well for sociological and political issues, such as "civil rights." For example, Stokeley Carmichael and George

Lincoln Rockwell judged the sociological adaptive value of the Black Muslim movement in radically different fashion. This cult's adaptive value for our *culture* will have to be judged historically, not psychoanalytically (no matter what might be our personal ethical, social, or political opinions). The psychological adaptive potential for this cult must be evaluated out of psychological data obtained from patients, not from one's own ethical, political, philosophical, or social views of this cryptic group. For the aforementioned homicidal Black Muslim patient, the sect was a psychologically adaptive (a la Hartmann) haven before, during, and after his acute schizophrenic episode. His beleaguered ego needed every bit of external control offered by his leader and his sect, as much as his superego required the communal sanction to hate the white man and even blame him for his "imprisonment" (hospitalization).

It must be restated that Freud's major works on religion, even though extrapolated and contributed to by his clinical observations, move well out of the range of analytic science on to his philosophy and his personal point of view. His idea that religion, as an illusion of the masses, serves as a preventive measure for individual neuroses is controvertible within the framework of psychoanalytic principles. (See "Future of an Illusion" [17], and compare these overgeneralizations with his statement [20], "For these ideas (theories) are not the foundation of science upon which everything rests: that foundation is observation alone.") First, with that word "masses" we already transported from individual scientific observation into the world of applied psychoanalysis and philosophical opinion at best. Second, analysis is an individual matter, and extrapolations and universalities such as symbolism become speculative unless confirmed by associative data. Third, in my experience, psychologically determined choices of aspects of organized religion may be the stage on which is acted out the individual's neurotic character, with or without overt symptomatology but not necessarily with internal character or developmental alteration. A neurotic or psychotic character may simply be playing out on religion's stage a conflict that can be understood easily with clinical examination. Going even further afield, Freud believed that religion vouchsafes believers to protection from neurosis "by removing their parental complex"! In terms of our earlier discussion, it is clear that displacement (transference, condensation, symbolization, or projection) but not *removal* appears as a possibility.

When Freud moves from his generalizations about religion to specific cases, however, psychoanalytic principles of scientific status become obvious. In regard to the "Wolfman," after carefully delineating a number of psychodynamic clarifications of his patient's religious cathexes, Freud added, "Apart from these pathological phenomena it may be said that in the present case religion achieved all the aims for the sake of which it is included in the education of the individual." It offered a restraint on his sexual impulsions "by affording a sublimation and a safe mooring." It lowered the importance of his patient's family directly, yet without isolation, through "access to the great community of mankind. The untamed and fear-ridden child became social, well-behaved, and amenable to education." His patient's identification with Christ brought Freud to conclude, "So it was that religion did its work for the hardpressed child by the combination which it afforded the believer of satisfaction, of sublimation, of diversion from sensual processes to purely spiritual ones, and of access to social relationships." These observations move us, most definitely, from symptomatic religious cathexes into the realm of the adaptive possibilities that systems of religion can afford the individual.

Hans Vaihinger [31] looked at the subject of fantasy and illusion, describing these phenomena in 1925 as "ficta." He noted the useful necessity of fictions as follows: "The 'As If' world, the world of the unreal,' is just as important as the world of the so-called real or actual; indeed, it is far more important for ethics and esthetics." He viewed a dogma as a "provisional auxiliary construction, necessary because the actual metaphysical relationship is incomprehensible." Of Schleiermacher's deity, he says, "God is not the 'Father of men' but He is to be treated and regarded *as if* He were." "Ficta" he regarded as never verifiable but "fused" with "reality" to provide useful hypotheses by which men live. (Nietzsche, too, points out that illusional concepts are to be considered a part of nature and must be understood to have both historical and psychological importance. He likened their importance to the importance of fairy tales and children's games in their contribution to survival.) [28]

Hartmann [21] saw adaptation as related to tasks of reality mastery, as a reciprocal relationship between the organism and its environment, favorable to its survival. He indicated that adaptation was guaranteed by man's primary equipment, the maturation of his mental apparatuses, and by ego-regulated actions that counteract the disturbances of the environment and at times alter them for the better. He elaborated on the importance of "fitting together" and the synthetic function of the ego that makes for internal equilibrium and keeping the peace between the three structures of the mind. In a much later paper [24], he observed that the ego's integration and adaptive capacities make the superego compatible with society and the self. Further, he pointed out that a moral system represents in different degrees the demands of the ego-ideal and the "ought not" of the superego.

In a world rocked by the fear of mass and individual violence, theologians have been challenged to find *new* adaptive resources in religion. As much as the individual psychological scientist might wish to maintain his own sense of a "Mysterium Tremendum" or, oppositely, feel the challenge to prove its illusion in others, his *investigatory* task requires purity from these biases. The avenues of the intrapsychological exploration of religion are still quiet, untrafficked lanes.

Why is religion such a powerful "stalking horse"? How does LSD stimulate "religious experiences"? Are there psychological explanations for their apparent similarities? Can "religious conversion" be harnessed for integrative use? Does religion blunt or prime creativity? Does it augment, facilitate, or challenge regression? What are its transitional object (Winnicott) possibilities? [33] Does it free the guilty or double-bind them? Does it simply reflect parental attitudes? Does it stifle or stimulate childhood development? Does a belief system mirror a healthy ego, help mold one, or need to be present to be outgrown or reacted against? Does it impoverish or broaden libidinal outlets? Does an external morality control violence or incite it? Does it cure or inhibit? Does it offer constructive or destructive myths? Does it matter at all?

Perhaps it is time we investigators of the mind took a second (and more objective) look at religious offerings that may have unrecognized progressive or regressive adaptational potency for our patients.

REFERENCES

1. Arlow, J. A. and Brenner, C. *Psychoanalytic Concepts and the Structural Theory.* New York: International Universities Press, 1964.
2. Brierley, M. Further notes on the implications of psychoanalysis: Metapsychology and personality. *Int. J. Psychoanal.* 26:106, 1945.
3. Carlson, H. Characteristics of an acute confusional state in college students. *Amer. J. Psychiat.* 114:900, 1958.
4. Christensen, C. W. Religious conversion. *Arch. Gen. Psychiat.* (Chicago) 9:207, 1963.
5. Draper, E. A metapsychological approach to religious data. *To be published.*
6. Draper, E. Religion as an intrapsychic experience. *Cinti. J. Med.* In press.
7. Draper, E., Meyer, G. G., Paren, Z., and Samuelson, G. On the diagnostic value of religious ideation. *Arch. Gen. Psychiat.* (Chicago) 13:202, 1965.
8. Eissler, K. R. Remarks on the psychoanalysis of schizophrenia. *Int. J. Psychoanal.* 32:18, 1951.
9. Freud, S. The Interpretation of Dreams (1903). In *The Complete Psychological Works of Sigmund Freud* (Std. ed.). London: Hogarth Press, 1955, Vol. V.
10. Freud, S. A Metapsychological Supplement to the Theory of Dreams. In *The Complete Psychological Works of Sigmund Freud* (Std. ed.). London: Hogarth Press, 1957, Vol. XIV, p. 226.
11. Freud, S. A Religious Experience. In *The Complete Psychological Works of Sigmund Freud* (Std. ed.). London: Hogarth Press, 1961, Vol. XXI, p. 167.
12. Freud, S. From the History of an Infantile Neurosis. In *The Complete Psychological Works of Sigmund Freud* (Std. ed.). London: Hogarth Press, 1955, Vol. XVII, p. 7.
13. Freud, S. Psychoanalytic Notes on an Autobiographical Account of a Case of Paranoia. In *The Complete Psychological*

Works of Sigmund Freud (Std. ed.). London: Hogarth Press, 1958, Vol. XII, p. 9.
14. Freud, S. Creative Writers and Day Dreaming. In *The Complete Psychological Works of Sigmund Freud* (Std. ed.). London: Hogarth Press, 1959, Vol. IX, p. 147.
15. Freud, S. Some Neurotic Mechanisms in Jealousy, Paranoia and Homosexuality. In *The Complete Psychological Works of Sigmund Freud* (Std. ed.). London: Hogarth Press, 1955, Vol. XVIII, p. 228.
16. Freud, S. Humour. In *The Complete Psychological Works of Sigmund Freud* (Std. ed.). London: Hogarth Press, 1961, Vol. XXI, p. 165.
17. Freud, S. The Future of an Illusion. In *The Complete Psychological Works of Sigmund Freud* (Std. ed.). London: Hogarth Press, 1961, Vol. XXI, p. 14.
18. Freud, S. Totem and Taboo. In *The Complete Psychological Works of Sigmund Freud* (Std. ed.). London: Hogarth Press, 1955, Vol. XIII, p. 1.
19. Freud, S. The Ego and the Id. In *The Complete Psychological Works of Sigmund Freud* (Std. ed.). London: Hogarth Press, 1961, Vol. XIX, p. 37.
20. Freud, S. On Narcissism. In *The Complete Psychological Works of Sigmund Freud* (Std. ed.). London: Hogarth Press, 1957, Vol. XIV, p. 77.
21. Hartmann, H. *Ego Psychology and the Problem of Adaptation.* New York: International Universities Press, 1958.
22. Hartmann, H. *Essays on Ego Psychology.* New York: International Universities Press, 1964.
23. Hartmann, H. The metapsychology of schizophrenia. *Psychoanal. Stud. Child* 8:177, 1953.
24. Hartmann, H., and Lowenstein, R. M. Notes on the superego. *Psychoanal. Stud. Child* 17:78, 1962.
25. Kohut, H. Introspection, empathy and psychoanalysis. *J. Amer. Psychoanal. Ass.* 7:459, 1959.
26. Kohut, H. Beyond the bound of the basic rule, some recent contributions to applied psychoanalysis. *J. Amer. Psychoanal. Ass.* 8:567, 1960.
27. Kris, E. On preconscious mental processes. *Psychoanal. Quart.* 19:557, 1950.
28. Nietzsche, Friedrich. Volumes III, IV, *Complete Works.* Edinburgh and London: T. N. Foulis, 1909-14.

29. Ostow, M. The need to believe. *Int. Rec. Med. Gen. Pract. Cl.* 168:798, 1955.
30. Rapaport, D., and Gill, M. The points of view and assumptions of metapsychology. *Int. J. Psychoanal.* 40:155, 1959.
31. Vaihinger, H. *The Philosophy of "As If."* New York: Harcourt, Brace, 1925.
32. Waelder, R. Psychoanalysis, scientific method and philosophy. *J. Amer. Psychoanal. Ass.* 10:617, 1962.
33. Winnicott, D. W. Transitional objects and transitional phenomena. *Int. J. Psychoanal.* 34:89, 1953.

The Existential Approach to Religion

CLEMENS E. BENDA

TWO VIEWS OF MAN

In a memorable dialogue between Freud and Binswanger, in Vienna in 1927, the two men discussed the fact that in some cases of psychoanalysis all insight is not sufficient to bring about a change in the patient and a recovery from his neurosis [9].

This exchange of ideas is so significant that it may serve as a starting point for the presentation of two opposing views that represent not only two different scientific approaches, but the dividing line of two eras in the understanding of man.

Binswanger [9] reports that, using a severe case of obsessional neurosis that had preoccupied both analysts as a clinical example, he raised the question of how we were to understand the failure of such a patient to take the last decisive step of psychoanalytical insight and become well. Instead, the patient persists in his misery, in defiance of all efforts and technical progress made so far. Binswanger suggested that such a failure may be understood as the result of something that could only be called a "lacking in spirituality" or the inability to reach the level of spiritual communication with his physician. Only from this vantage point can the needed insight into certain unconscious drives be attained and the patient become able to take the last decisive step toward "overcoming his self-centered-

37

ness" (die Selbstüberwindung) or, as we may say today, toward
transcendence. Binswanger continues: "I could hardly believe my
ears when I heard Freud say: 'Yes, spirit is everything.' " Binswanger
thought that by "spirit" Freud meant something like intelligence,
but Freud continued to say that "mankind has always known that
it possesses spirit: I had to show that there are also drives (instincts)."

Binswanger went on to say, "encouraged by this admission, I went
a step further, explaining that I found myself forced to recognize in
man something like a basic religious category. In any case it was
impossible for me to admit that the religious was a phenomenon
that could somehow be derived from something else. (I was thinking, of course, not of the origin of a particular religion, nor even of
a religion in general, but of something that I have since learned to
call the religious I-thou relationship.)" Binswanger continues:

> I had stretched the bow of agreement too far and began to feel its
> resistance. "Religion originates in the helplessness and anxiety of
> childhood and early manhood," Freud curtly said. "It cannot be
> otherwise."
> With that, he went to the drawer of his desk: "This is the moment
> for me to show you something," and he laid down before me a
> completed manuscript that bore the title "The Future of an Illu-
> sion" [13].
> He looked at me with an inquiring smile. From the trend of our
> conversation I easily guessed what the title meant. It was time for
> me to go. Freud walked with me to the door. His last words, spoken
> with a shrewd, slightly ironic smile, were: "I am sorry I cannot
> satisfy your religious needs."
> Never was it more difficult for me to take leave of my great and
> revered friend than it was at that moment when, in full awareness
> of the "great idea" that culminated his gigantic struggle and had
> come to be his destiny, he held out his hand to me.

Space does not allow us to go into any further detail about Freud's
ideas about religion, which he has amplified in "The Future of an
Illusion." Suffice it to say that very few people realize that Freud's
statements about religion—such as the one quoted above, that religion originates in the helplessness and anxiety of childhood and
early manhood, or his more definite pronouncement from "The
Future of an Illusion," that religion is the general human compul-

sive neurosis that originates, like that of children, from the Oedipus complex—all these statements have nothing to do with religion and are, at best, psychological observations indicating why some people are religious and other people may not be. Freud's statements do not indicate any scientific insight and are just as weak and prejudiced as the statement of Karl Marx, "Religion is opium for the people," made one hundred years earlier, or the writings of the philosopher Feuerbach [11, 12], who developed all those ideas that Freud used in "The Future of an Illusion" in the middle of the nineteenth century.

THE ISSUE OF FREEDOM

What is touched upon in this famous dialogue between Freud and Binswanger is a problem that has intrigued countless psychotherapists, and also educators, ministers, and all people who are concerned with the welfare of man. We see that the last decisive step in psychoanalysis is to extricate the patient from the captivity of his neurosis and make him a free person. We agree that the patient cannot extricate himself or pull himself up by his own bootstraps. Although some people may consider a neurosis a weakness and blame the patient, the majority of intelligent people will not fall back into those medieval views, but will acknowledge that the patient needs help. The patient himself, as a patient, recognizes his own inability to extricate himself, and he is inspired by the hope that psychoanalysis will do this work for him. Moreover, many patients will say, "If I only could believe, if I could have faith, if I could commit myself to anything, I would be well."

In the dialogue between Freud and Binswanger, both psychiatrists admit that psychoanalysis as such is, in certain cases, not able to do the job either, and the patient remains in the prison of his neurosis. Freud as a rationalist is willing to admit this failure and considers it a kind of lack of rationality that prevents the severely neurotic, compulsive patient from liberating himself from his unconscious, irrational hang-ups, joining the community of rational

people, and acting in a predictable and intelligent manner. Binswanger, as a younger man, is able to see beyond Freud's rationality
and, being on the doorstep of a new century, the era of "irrational
man," Binswanger realizes that something else is necessary to extricate man from his neurosis. He tentatively calls this force religion, or we may also say it is love or the I-thou relationship.

Before we enter into a discussion of what is meant here by the
phenomenon of religion or spirit, a brief remark may be made with
regard to the problem of curing the compulsive neurotic who is unable to transcend his own captivity.

In the years between the famous dialogue and the present time,
a wealth of material has come to light that indicates that the hysterical patient, who was such a successful subject of psychoanalytical treatment, still belongs and is a part of a loving relationship,
even if in rebellion and using abnormal routes of escape. But the
compulsive neurotic and obsessive is the alienated man who does
not belong and does not want to belong. There is no inducement to
leave one's own isolation, and the self-preservation of one's own
lonely individuality is preferable to giving up one's ego defenses in
favor of something that is not one's own. The problem of improvement and cure of compulsive neurosis cannot be approached any-
more from the viewpoint of lack of spirituality or lack of religion.
Thus, Freud is perfectly justified in saying that conventional religion does not provide means for liberating the patient from his
predicament.

RELIGION AS AN ORIENTATION

As we now proceed to analyze the phenomenon of religion, we
are not investigating a specific form of institutionalized religion;
rather, we are dealing with the phenomenon of religion as it appears in the religious experience of all man. Whatever the definition
of religion is, whether we believe with Cicero that the word "religion" is related to the Latin root *leg*, which would indicate the
action of collecting or observing—meaning that religion is "the

reading of the divine signs and revelations"—or we assume with Servius that religion is related to the Latin root *lig,* which means binding—implying that religion is the relationship of man to the divine—there is no question that religion is the orientation of man toward those aspects of life that transcend the present. Religious questions deal with life and death, illness and health, judgment and justification, and, thus, with a way of life, with behavior, and, therefore, with morality, responsibility, and actions that may be justifiable before the strictest standards of conscience. From an individualistic point of view, morality—and all morality is rooted in religion—is merely an inhibiting factor that limits the individual freedom. Man can, at best, adjust to the unavoidable. From a rationalist's point of view, religion is the irrational, unscientific, emotional reaction to the unexplainable aspects of life, a reaction that is unrealistic, neurotic, immature, and will eventually yield to the progress of a more enlightened humanity [15].

From an existential, phenomenological point of view, individualism and rationalism are "isms" that misunderstand man's being in the world and the predicament of his existence.

First of all, man is a social being. Whether he likes it or not, he is dependent on others. His world is shaped by others and he lives in a complex network of interrelationships. His social existence makes him interact with others, and others depend on him. Any social interaction rests on mutuality, predictability, responsibilities, and commitment [8]. One cannot step out, unpunished, from the roles that one has accepted and that one must play to maintain the social community.

These fundamental data force the study of religion to recognize certain ontological facts. Man, as a being, is confronted with a world; he faces his existence as something that he has not created, but that he experiences, that acts upon him, influences him, in short, moves him like the wind moves the trees. It is for this reason that all languages are inspired to express the experience of the spiritual by the metaphor of breath (*spirare*), as indicated by such words as inspiration, expiration, and aspiration.

Being exposed to the world to which we belong, we find that this

world is not a reality that is the same for all. Since each individual
is confronted with the world from a different stand in space and
time (geneticists state that no two human beings of the world population have the same fundamental genetic coding), no two human
beings perceive the world in the same way. Each individual experiences existence in a different way, according to his own position, and
thus he perceives, selects, and responds to being in the world in his
own way. Last, but not least, man's being is *becoming*. He is not
completed from the very beginning, but rather is in a state of constant transformation that is not, like physical development and
aging, merely a passive event; it is a matter of choices and decisions
that increasingly become man's responsibility, to which he may
respond or which he may avoid [6].

We shall not deal here with phenomenology in more detail [1, 2].
Given the few fundamentals above, it goes without saying that the
phenomenological approach to religion is an entirely different one.
Religion must be viewed as man's most fundamental endeavor to
organize human morality in a way that not only covers temporary
laws and conveniences, codes and customs, but makes man a being
who thinks and acts in human terms rather than as a member of a
specific nation, race, tribe, or creed. To transcend man's temporality
and serve humanity in a lasting way beyond a given space and
time requires concepts of lasting truth, ultimate concern, convic-
tions, commitments, and responsibilities that are not judged by
one's contemporaries or their courts (who may even contradict their
own decisions with each new political appointment). Man's conscience is rooted in the idea of justification [8], the idea that man
could stand judgment by a God who transcends space and time,
who is "eternal," and who judges man by standards that are neither
provincial nor local in human terms.

However imperfect all human religions are or have been, however unsatisfactory and childish man's aspirations may be, to achieve
anything lasting and universal from his limited, relative, and
basically agnostic position, it is obvious that none of the voiced
criticism of religion has any ontological significance. All such pro-

nouncements only reveal the inadequacy of any temporary formulation of a religious interpretation of the world.

DEVOTION AND DEDICATION

If we try now to view the fundamental phenomenon that constitutes religion, we must acknowledge that religion is not a certain belief, but that aspect of living to which one's being is devoted. As Erwin Ramsdell Goodenough [14] pointed out, "We cannot define religion by saying that it is the worship of God or the gods, but we can define God or the gods by saying they are whatever is the object of devotion." And he continues, rather resignedly: "Most just plug along in polytheistic devotion to science, money, metaphysical dreams, family, social success, and what not."

We must recognize that, in facing the world, man is confronted with vast areas of being, which he cannot understand, of which he has very incomplete knowledge, and which he cannot control; all living involves the constant coding and ordering of experience, in order to provide security, mutual dependability, and goal-directed action. In being, life itself is the great mystery. What life is worth living? Mere survival, mere existence is not enough. The psychiatrist who deals with the inner life of man is constantly confronted with the facts that life without meaning is not worth living and that each individual strives toward being devoted and dedicated to something greater than himself.

Devotion and dedication represent value choices. As I have emphasized several times, values are not superimposed, additional evaluations above a primarily value-free mode of existence; value choices are intrinsic to living itself. No being could survive without the ability to select and reject and to commit himself to one mode of action that necessarily excludes all other routes available at the same time. Ralph W. Burhoe [10] reminded us recently of the notion set forth by Erwin Schrödinger [20] and Norbert Wiener [22], that the evolution of life is a program that runs exactly counter to the general or most probable program of the surrounding environment. Burhoe says, "Evolving life is the growth of organization or order which represents a decrease in entropy in a world that in general operates . . . in the direction of increasing entropy or increasing disorder." Schrödinger [20] says: "A living organism has the astonishing gift of concentrating a *stream of order* on itself and thus escaping the decay into atomic chaos—in *drinking orderliness* from a suitable environment."

MORALITY AND RELIGION

The living forms are organized by genetic coding, and the biological world of the animal kingdom is regulated by instincts, but man's social organism is not provided with definite rules and codes that are binding for all. The morality of each culture is centered around a central theme [16], which attempts to formulate human existence in terms that are all-embracing and transcend the needs and wishes of smaller privileged groups who desire to use religion as a defense for their own selfish interests. Therefore, while each religion tries to base its morality on lasting, divine commandments, religion by its very nature does not permit the abuse of God for selfish reasons, and each religion provides, at the same time, the spiritual forces that overcome stagnation and the righteousness of those who claim divine privileges. The very fact that all great religions defy man's temporality by measuring man's life by timeless, "eternal" standards (in Buddhism man's time is an illusion, in Christianity a second measured by eternity) has prodded religious people through all centuries to revolt in the name of conscience [8] and to attempt time and again a new formulation of the Divine.

As a social being, man needs a moral order. Since much order is only meaningful if it has lasting value, the individual will only recognize the immediacy and urgency of any such postulate if he feels assured that the powers who try to enforce their rules are serving higher powers and not their self-interest, and if to obey such commandments has a meaning for the individual's life. By life we mean here not being alive and seeking pleasure and fulfillment, but life seen in the perspective of life and death, in the perspective of having to account for one's deeds and emerge justified. Although modern man's ideas about a last judgment may be rather vague, and many may prefer not to think of it at all, even the so-called atheistic existentialism recognizes the need of an "authentic" life, and rejects a living that lacks individuality and neglects to accept the Karma of each life.

THE ROLE OF THE PSYCHIATRIST

The modern psychiatrist should be able to treat people of all races and creeds. The reintroduction of concepts such as sin into psychology and psychiatry [18, 21] appears to this writer very unfortunate, and the idea of a "religious or Christian psychiatrist" seems a contradiction in itself. But psychiatry has to recognize that patients or clients in need are not only individuals with a psychic apparatus that could be repaired; they are beings who operate in a world of human interrelationships and cultural currents that have formed them and that form the framework of their thinking.

Space does not permit me to go into much detail here, but a few striking examples may be touched upon. The central theme of western civilization has been crystallized around the Hellenistic-Judaic-Christian interpretation of man's life and role. We are now confronted with a growing hostility and violence that is bound to disrupt the whole social organism. The neurotic of our time is reared in a "fatherless," loveless, and often emotionally deprived childhood, the terror of which only the psychoanalytically trained psychiatrist can fathom. Psychoanalysis believes that the incessant return to childhood experiences may wear out the intensity of the hate and resentment that was generated in those years and is now rekindled. Does the flame of hate and revenge really burn out by itself? Western religion has provided the concept of forgiveness. Without entering into a discussion of the sacral implications that require man to forgive to be forgiven, is the concept of forgiving not a psychological-spiritual force that enables the person to permit injustice and insult to be forgotten [19]? The study of creativity [4] makes it very clear that man's creative life depends as much on what can be forgotten, what can be eradicated, as on what is remembered and incorporated.

A central concept of western thinking is that of love and sacrifice. Modern man has become almost allergic to these ideas. Because he is reared in a selfish, loveless world, postulates such as selflessness and selfless love have an ironical and cynical sound to modern man. Yet the phenomenological approach to being reveals clearly that the individual is always suspended between the urgent immediacy of his bodily needs—his drives, desires, and appetites—and the otherness of the world, which is not composed of drive-objects and things to be subjected to man's aggressive and destructive actions, but rather is peopled by other human beings of equal value and dignity [5].

Religious transcendence is the ability to see one's own feelings and thoughts in the context of the greater community to which we belong. Religion reminds people that they are creatures among others. If they demand to be loved, they must subjugate their isolated existence to a community of men with whom they share. In the language of religious tradition, what appears so foreign to modern ears is nothing but the insight that you cannot serve mankind without serving an image of God, who represents those aspects of Nature that are not rooted in selfish interests and fulfillment of biological needs. The greatest fulfillment is found in a creative endeavor that transcends the present and stands the test of time.

We have indicated that religion is concerned with Time. To emancipate human life from the evanescence of being in its constant flux of fleeting emotions and thoughts and subordinate it into an order that has duration and lasting value has been the concern of all religious thought. The Western world has increasingly formed the image of God in visual images that are spacial and static by nature. God is "seen" and visualized in terms of "above" or "within." The theology of the death of God is the funeral rites of a god who is static and not able to reign over the immensity of the cosmic space. Man has forgotten that God is invisible. The dimension of God is time. God speaks through time. Mankind's obsession to form visual images of all thoughts prevents most people from forming a nonvisual image that has "substance" like a melody [5] and yet has no bodily model. The God of religion is "timeless" because He speaks only through time.

REFERENCES

1. Benda, C. E.   The existential approach in psychiatry. *J. Exist. Psychiat.* 1:24, 1960.
2. Benda, C. E.   Existentialism in philosophy and science. *J. Exist. Psychiat.* 1:284, 1960.
3. Benda, C. E.   Emotions and freedom of will. *J. Lib. Ministry* 2:49, 1962.
4. Benda, C. E.   Language, intelligence, and creativity. *J. Exist. Psychiat.* 3:28, 1962.
5. Benda, C. E.   *The Image of Love.* New York: Free Press, 1961.
6. Benda, C. E.   What is existential psychiatry? *Amer. J. Psychiat.* 123:288, 1966.
7. Benda, C. E.   Neuroses of conscience. *J. Exist. Psychiat.* 7:125, 1967.
8. Benda, C. E.   *The Troubled Conscience: Psychiatric, Religious and Political Aspects of Guilt.* In press.
9. Binswanger, L.   *Being-in-the-World* (trans. J. Needleman). New York: Basic Books, 1963.
10. Burhoe, R. W.   Five steps in the evolution of man's knowledge of good and evil. *Zygon, J. Relig. Sci.* 2:77, 1967.
11. Feuerbach, Ludwig.   *Das Wesen des Christentums.* Leipzig, 1841.
12. Feuerbach, Ludwig.   *Das Wesen der Religion.* Leipzig, 1851.
13. Freud, Sigmund.   The Future of an Illusion (1927). In *The Complete Psychological Works of Sigmund Freud* (Std. ed.). London: Hogarth Press, 1961, Vol. XXI.
14. Goodenough, E. R.   A historian of religion tries to define religion. *Zygon, J. Relig. Sci.* 2:7, 1967.
15. Greenson, Ralph.   The Conflict Between Religion and Psychoanalysis, Lecture, quoted by E. M. Pattison in Ego morality: An emerging psychotherapeutic concept. *Psychoanal. Rev.* 52:187, 1968.

16. Kluckhohn, C. Introduction. In W. A. Lessa and E. Z. Vogt (Eds.), *Reader in Comparative Religion: An Anthropological Approach* (2nd ed.). New York: Harper & Row, 1966.
17. Laing, R. D. *The Divided Self.* London: Tavistock, 1963.
18. Mowrer, O. H. *The Crisis in Psychiatry and Religion.* Princeton, N.J.: Van Nostrand, 1961.
19. Pattison, E. M. Ego morality: An emerging psychotherapeutic concept. *Psychoanal. Rev.* 52:187, 1968.
20. Schrödinger, Erwin. *What Is Life?* New York: Doubleday, 1956.
21. Tournier, P. *The Strong and the Weak.* Philadelphia: Westminster, 1963.
22. Wiener, N. *The Human Use of Human Beings.* Boston: Houghton Mifflin, 1950.

A Psychoanalytic View of Religion

ALBERT J. LUBIN

A boy was born while a blazing comet passed near the earth. His deeply religious parents, devout members of a Fundamentalist church, regarded this as a sign from God of his special nature and named him David, after the Old Testament hero. At the age of three, the boy, who had been jealous of his father, stirred up an argument between his parents, in the midst of which his father dropped dead of apoplexy. He inferred that he was responsible for the death and thereafter became terrified that he could mysteriously kill off big people. In the course of his religious training, he came to regard himself as David the Giant Killer, a self-image that eventually enabled him to channel hostility into socially acceptable paths. As an adult he devoted many of his resources to defeating giant corporations, a diversion of his feared killer instincts that helped him become a successful, honorable, and respected professional man. There were also other aspects to this self-image. For instance, he once observed a beautiful young woman sunning herself beside the pool of the resort where he was vacationing. She wore a flesh-colored, clinging swim suit and a wedding ring. He soon stole her from her husband and for many years kept her as his mistress. True to his destiny, a destiny that was quite unknown to him, he had acquired his Bathsheba. Only during the course of psychoanalysis did he become aware that he had been acting out the role of the Biblical David in many and diverse forms.

49

Psychologists have tended to consider religion on the basis of its effect on human character and human behavior. At the turn of the century, William James [14] claimed that religion should be judged by its impact on behavior. Wilhelm Wundt [25], a contemporary who was otherwise critical of James' pragmatic approach, seems to have concurred with this idea. The case of David is an example of the use of religious images in finding solutions to life's problems, albeit not in the way that churchmen might anticipate. Even though he had not been affiliated with a church since he was a youngster, David's behavior—indeed, his whole life pattern—was influenced by his religious background. But it was the kind of cause-and-effect relation that ordinary observation, psychiatric examination, and psychological testing failed to reveal.

This illustrates the difficulty in determining and evaluating the results of exposure to religious phenomena. Father Godin [10] points out that religious education functions without reference to its demonstrated effectiveness; that not one published study has taken for its object the evaluation of the influence of a method of religious instruction. He discusses three difficulties in evaluating the relation between church and behavior [11]: (1) Observable behavior is ambiguous; knowledge of man's inner feelings and thoughts is needed in order to know behavior's full meaning. (2) Motivations toward religious belonging are often overdetermined, and attitudes toward religion are partly conscious, partly unconscious. (3) Ambivalence about religious attitudes (i.e., twofold affective tendencies such as sympathy and antagonism, fascination and terror, and participation and rejection) and identifications with both a loved model (such as Christ) and with the church community must be considered.

These ideas are derived from the psychoanalytic point of view, a view that stresses the contribution of the unconscious mind, the mental coexistence of opposites, and the complex nature of human thoughts, emotions, and behavior. It recognizes that man is usually motivated from different directions at the same time. A religious influence may simultaneously mollify the conscience, gratify the instincts, and be a vehicle for adaptation. The need to satisfy id, ego, and superego alike makes the so-called principle of multiple function a necessity, not an accident.

Furthermore, religion is but one of the agencies that influence man, and the various influences may be difficult to disentangle. Such diverse forces as the Boy Scouts, television drama, and comic books, as well as political, economic, and geographic factors, each compete with religion for a place in the psychic economy. When the religious idea and the psychic life of the individual have some special affinity (as in the case of any of these influences), brief or seemingly casual exposure to the idea may influence development more profoundly than frequent and prolonged exposure under different circumstances. In addition, ideas that are irrelevant to the religious message may be as significant in influencing character as the religious doctrines themselves. For example, a Methodist whose life was profoundly influenced by John Wesley, the founder of Methodism, assumed many personal traits of Wesley that were unrelated to his religion [8]. These included interests in scholarly activity, foreign languages, and editing, as well as arising before dawn and keeping a daily journal. The technique of psychoanalysis is the method that is particularly suited to studying the extremely variegated and dynamic meanings of behavior derived from religious inculcation.

The basic contributions to the psychoanalytic study of religion have come from Freud, although recent theoretical advances have increased their range and promise. Perhaps Freud's two most challenging contributions in this area were in "Totem and Taboo" (1911) [6] and "The Future of an Illusion" (1927) [7]. The first was primarily a study of the origin of religion, and the second a study of its nature. In "Totem and Taboo" Freud concluded that God was formed in the likeness of an exalted father and that religion had its origin in a primeval Oedipus complex. In "The Future of an Illusion," Freud suggested that religions, "in their psychological nature," were illusions (i.e., beliefs based primarily on wish-fulfillment). Man is driven to them by his helplessness in the face of danger: the dangers of nature, the fear of death, the need to relieve the

suffering that society imposes on man. Although Freud stated that
psychoanalysis was "neither religious nor its opposite," his atheistic
bias sometimes influenced his point of view and, in the case of the
Wolf-Man, his therapeutic endeavors [21].

Recent advances in psychoanalysis have, on one side, been concerned with the first year of life and the role of the pre-oedipal
mother. As a result, the maternal aspects of God images have been
seen more clearly [17]. On the other side, psychoanalysis has come to
recognize more fully the workings of adaptive and creative processes
and the complex interrelation between man and society. Hartmann
[12], one of the leading Freudian theoreticians, has said:

The continued influence on the human mind and the synthetic
achievement of religions rest on their integrative imagery and on
their being tradition-saturated, socially unifying wholes which are
fed by the contributions of all three mental institutions [id, ego,
superego] and provide a pattern accessible to many people for satisfying the demands of all three institutions. . . . Religions are the
most obvious attempt to cope both with these mental institutions
and with social adaptation (through forming communities) by means
of synthesis.

Erikson has applied his contributions on identity formation to
studying the effects of religion on development in *Young Man
Luther* [4]. His schema concerning the psychosocial aspects of the
developmental stages (in which basic trust, for instance, is treated
as the outcome of a satisfactory progression through the early oral-
sensory stage) [3] and the basic virtues to be derived from each stage
(hope, will power, purpose, competence, fidelity, care, and wisdom)
[5] open the way for continued psychoanalytic and sociological research. One may postulate, for example, that (1) religion can serve
many functions, from the most primitive psychological needs to the
most complex integrative patterns, for both the individual and the
group; (2) it can serve these perpetually evolving functions during
all of Erikson's psychosexual and psychosocial stages of development and influence the outcome of each stage; and (3) it can reinforce, modify, or reverse at later periods the original outcome of
each developmental stage and thereby influence future stages. These

postulates could then be tested by studying the effects of various religious elements (e.g., communion) in terms of Erikson's criteria. Does a particular element assist or hinder the development of the stage in which it occurs and the stages to follow? Is it capable of modifying the outcome of previous stages? Such studies are yet to be undertaken.

Psychoanalysis has its own sphere of competence, limited by its techniques and by the type of data it accumulates: (1) As a time-consuming procedure aimed at understanding the complex variables in each person rather than searching for shared factors among groups of people, its ability to compile statistics or to prove its hypotheses using statistical methods is extremely limited. (2) A behavior pattern or symptom can be traced to its source in the mind but cannot be predicted from knowledge of these sources. Similarly, psychoanalysis can analyze the various basic psychological components of a ritual, for instance, but it cannot reverse the situation and predict the development of the ritual from these same components [8]. Psychosocial processes are far too complicated for that. (3) While psychoanalysis may make judgments on the efficacy of religions in combating fear or guilt [22] or reveal their contributions to attitudes and behavior, it cannot gauge the moral worth of these effects. (4) Finally, psychoanalysis cannot deal with the reality or unreality of transcendental phenomena, although it may reveal how they are put to psychological use. It can neither prove nor disprove the "true" nature of such ideas as God, revelation, or grace. In spite of the transparency of this statement, some psychologically trained theologians attempt to prove the presence of these phenomena by combining psychoanalysis and theology, and some psychoanalysts pronounce negative value judgments on theological issues that are outside the ken of their discipline.

A full exposition of the psychoanalytic meaning of religious belief, if such were possible, would be as complicated and far-ranging as an explanation of the mind itself, with all its reciprocal, overlapping conflict-solving and adaptive dynamisms, as well as its relation to the function of social systems. From a psychological point of view, religion may alleviate fears of destruction, loss, and death;

control instinctual drives; pattern stimuli inducing shame and guilt, as well as provide for their relief; and establish uniform models of defense and adaptation. All but the first serve the purposes of the group more than those of the individual, and from this standpoint religions act as legal or paternalistic systems. But they may also be capable of inducing states of mind that contribute to self-realization and of aiding their believers in arriving at an ideology that will enable them to carry on their heritage while at the same time giving them meaningful goals for their anticipated future.

Psychoanalysts or psychoanalytically oriented psychotherapists who are alert to the religious allusions made by their patients will accumulate a large amount of data concerning the use and effect of these allusions. One might argue that religious ideation influences everything, or almost everything, that some patients communicate. Manifest references to religion occur in about one-third of all psychoanalytic sessions [8]. In addition, numerous thoughts, words, and gestures that are not obviously "religious" are disguised derivatives. A beckoning hand motion assumed by a patient when he wished to obtain information from the analyst or other acquaintances, for instance, turned out to be an imitation of the priest of his childhood who beckoned him to the confessional in order to hear him document his sins.

The clinician who is aware of the relevance of religious themes to his work can make a variety of observations:

(1) He may correlate religious themes with the patient's symptoms, recalling, however, that such explanations are only partial. After traveling through desert country, a woman drove to the top of a mountain and looked into the lush valley below. There on the mountain she experienced a severe panic in which she feared she was dying. Psychoanalytic study showed that she was reliving a traumatic childhood experience; but at the same time she was reenacting the role of Moses who ascended Mount Nebo after years of wandering in the desert and looked into the Promised Land, only to die before reaching it [18]. Vincent van Gogh's mutilation of his own ear is another example [20]. The scene in Gethsemane, in which Simon

Peter cuts off the ear of the man who had come to seize Christ, was on van Gogh's mind prior to the self-mutilation. It is likely that he reenacted the scene when he cut off his ear.

Obsessional symptoms may be frank repetitions of religious rituals, as in the case of Freud's Wolf-Man [21], who repeated the Russian Orthodox priest's ritual at the iconostasis. Another man with obsessional symptoms, without being aware of it, converted the top of his bureau into a modified altar and feigned a modified mass each night before retiring.

(2) The clinician may find that the patient uses religious ideas to bolster his defenses. For example, the woman who reenacted the role of Moses had seen herself since childhood as low, dirty, and shameful. Being a fantasied Moses neutralized these uncomfortable feelings and helped her feel proud. The patient who imitated the beckoning motion of the priest was thereby transformed from an ignominious sinner who feared being shamed and punished into an agent of God who could shame and punish others. Some patients make a haloed God out of the therapist as a defense against fears of sexual or murderous impulses toward him.

(3) The clinician may also discover the psychological stresses and needs that precipitate a sudden religious conversion or, on the other hand, a virulent antireligious attitude. A turn to religion, for instance, may result from painful feelings of isolation, loss, and hopelessness that accompany a depressive episode. Faith in a mighty God and the fantasy of being united with Him may bring solace to the sufferer.

A different motivation was present in a 13-year-old girl who suddenly became fanatically religious and whose thoughts became preoccupied with a benevolent God in heaven. The increased sexual feelings of puberty had forced her to turn against her previously adored father as a protection against recurring incestuous wishes. One day, while alone in the country, she imagined that a white cloud became transformed into the face of God, and she felt safe and protected. The cloud God was an asexual father, far beyond her reach.

Sometimes the image of God becomes intertwined with childhood terrors. Scientific thinking may then be used to rationalize atheism and repress frightening religious ideation.

(4) The clinician may be able to clarify the influence of religion on the complex integrative processes involved in identity formation [16, 18, 19, 21]. This is a subject too extensive for a brief review. Hence I will restrict the discussion to two psychological mechanisms that are important in the process: identification and regression induced by the ritual.

Identification with a religious figure is one of the most common and effective ways in which religion influences personality and is a frequent element in adult identity formation. To quote from a previous essay [19]:

It is, perhaps, not too surprising that a Christian should identify himself with Christ and a Jew with Moses. Each is exposed to these awesome figures from an early age, figures who are held up as ideals to be revered and emulated. To be a good Christian is to be Christlike. But to be Christlike may mean something different to the child than to the adult. . . . Thus the outcome·of an identification with Christ may appear to the casual observer anything but Christlike.

Identifications with religious figures assume many garbs, for religious figures are perceived in different ways by different people, especially in childhood. The nature of the perception depends largely on the self-image of the perceiver and on those aspects of religious figures that serve as models for the resolution of conflict [1]. They may, however, be more than mere projections, more than a means of promoting previously acquired self-images. New qualities may be perceived in them that fill particular needs at crucial periods, and introjecting these qualities may add a new essence to living. They may also influence the whole personality development and play a part in determining work, sexual, and social patterns, even when the individual has consciously forsaken the gods and prophets of his childhood. They may act as bridges between the earliest identifications and self-images, many of which would be useless or harmful in real life, and the more or less completed identity of late adolescence or early adulthood.

In Western society Christ is undoubtedly the figure most often used as an object for identification; this is encouraged by partaking of the Eucharist during the mass. Identification with Christ may occur in such varied guises as (1) Christ as a suffering victim, ever seeking a Judas (seen among moral masochists); (2) Christ as an omniscient creator (seen in creative artists and scientists); (3) Christ as an aggressive hero on a white horse, making decisions of life and death (seen in a social worker); (4) Christ as a healer (seen in a physician); (5) Christ as a helpless Lamb of God (who loves to sing, "Who's Afraid of the Big Bad Wolf?"); (6) Christ as a masochistic homosexual (seen in a former Catholic who, as a boy, was sexually stimulated by the beatings of Christ on the Way of the Cross) [19]; (7) Christ as a paranoid personality who feels tricked and mistreated (observed among members of a Catholic church in a poor, mistreated town) [13]; and (8) Christ as a con man (seen in the "Hoodlum Priest," who works with murderers and thieves, explaining, "Christ was a con, too").

Ritual is one of the important means by which religion may influence man. Using prayer, music, chanting, distinctive dress, special postures, and other unusual or mysterious effects in a highly stylized ceremony, it creates, according to Max Weber [24], a "religious mood"; Weber considered this mood to be the "instrument of salvation." Awe, a state Otto [23] has described as the specific religious feeling, is one of its important components. Factors that facilitate the establishment of the religious mood include group identification during church worship, the psychological effect of church architecture (e.g., being inside the Mother Church), faith in the mysterious powers of the church, a filial relation to God or other religious figures (as well as an identification with them), and special techniques that divert attention and perception [2, 9] (akin to sensory isolation).

Reactivating the illogical, nondiscursive, magical thinking of childhood, ritual may generate a regression to earlier development phases that shares some features of the regression generated by the technique of psychoanalysis. Although some avoid it due to fear of psychological disintegration, the depth, intensity, and duration of the process is held under control by the ritual itself, except in orgiastic rituals that are permitted or encouraged to run wild. The depth of the regressive processes varies with the nature of the ritual and the motivation of the participant. The rather lighthearted ceremonies observed in some Sunday church meetings, where the minds of many participants are barely engaged in the ritual, can hardly be expected to achieve the same result as the intense, supervised daily meditation practices of Zen Buddhism, regardless of the underlying theological virtues of each.

The stimulation of regressive states may promote a fixation with infantile thinking, a faith in magic that is not tempered by rational thought, or the production of disorganized pathological states. Controlled regression, however, may be an enriching experience, the "regression in the service of the ego" that Kris [15] has described. The individual may experience a feeling of union with God, an adult version of the infantile state when the baby cannot differentiate between himself and his mother, and a symbolic rebirth may follow. Such deeply regressed states may be transient experiences in which the somatic or mental aspects of the self are temporarily transformed, or they may result in a reorganization of the personality that contributes to the developmental process as well as to productive and creative activity.

REFERENCES

1. Arlow, J. A. The consecration of the prophet. *Psychoanal. Quart.* 20:374, 1951.
2. Deikman, A. J. De-automatization and the mystic experience. *Psychiatry* 29:324, 1966.
3. Erikson, E. H. *Identity, Youth and Crisis.* New York: Norton, 1968.
4. Erikson, E. H. *Young Man Luther.* New York: Norton, 1958.
5. Erikson, E. H. Human Strength and the Cycle of Generations. In *Insight and Responsibility.* New York: Norton, 1964.
6. Freud, S. Totem and Taboo (1913). In *The Complete Psy-*

chological Works of Sigmund Freud (Std. ed.). London: Hogarth Press, 1955, Vol. XIII.

7. Freud, S. The Future of an Illusion (1927). In *The Complete Psychological Works of Sigmund Freud* (Std. ed). London: Hogarth Press, 1961, Vol. XXI.
8. The psychic function of religion in mental illness and health. *Group Advance. Psychiat.* [*Rep.*] 67, 1968.
9. Gill, M. M. and Brenman, M. *Hypnosis and Related States: Psychoanalytic Studies in Regression.* New York: International Universities Press, 1959.
10. Godin, A. Importance and Difficulty of Scientific Research in Religious Education: The Problem of the "Criterion." In S. W. Cook (Ed.), *Review of Recent Research Bearing on Religions and Character Formation.* New York: Religious Research Association, 1962.
11. Godin, A. Belonging to a Church: What Does It Mean Psychologically? *J. Sci. Stud. Relig.* 3:204, 1964.
12. Hartmann, H. *Ego Psychology and the Problem of Adaptation.* New York: International Universities Press, 1958.
13. Higgins, J. W. Personal communications, 1966.
14. James, W. *Varieties of Religious Experience.* New York: Longmans, Green, 1902.
15. Kris, E. *Psychoanalytic Explorations in Art.* New York: International Universities Press, 1952.
16. Leavy, S. A. Clinical observations on the development of religion in later childhood. *Bull. Phila. Assn. Psychoanal.* 11:61, 1961.
17. Loewald, H. Ego and reality. *Int. J. Psychoanal.* 32:10, 1951.
18. Lubin, A. J. A feminine Moses, a bridge between childhood identifications and adult identity. *Int. J. Psychoanal.* 39:535, 1958.
19. Lubin, A. J. A boy's view of Jesus. *Psychoanal. Stud. Child* 14:155, 1959.
20. Lubin, A. J. Vincent van Gogh's ear. *Psychoanal. Quart.* 30:351, 1961.
21. Lubin, A. J. The influence of the Russian Orthodox Church on Freud's Wolf-Man: A hypothesis (with an epilogue based on visits with the Wolf-Man). *Psychoanal. Forum* 2:145, 1967, and 2:281, 1967.
22. Ostow, M., and Scharfstein, B. *The Need to Believe.* New York: International Universities Press, 1954.

23. Otto, R. *The Idea of the Holy*. London: Oxford University Press, 1923.
24. Weber, M. *The Sociology of Religion*. Boston: Beacon Press, 1963.
25. Wundt, W. *Elements of Folk Psychology*. New York: Macmillan, 1916.

Pathological Processes in Religion

PHILIP WOOLLCOTT, JR.

INTRODUCTION

Most psychiatric studies of religious behavior, beginning with Freud [3], have traditionally focused on pathology, a fact that has raised the hackles of many religionists. But those who object to religious behavior's being examined primarily from the viewpoint of psychopathology should recall that our present knowledge of the psychology of "normal" behavior was derived primarily from efforts to understand mentally sick persons.

This report is a contribution to the study of religious experience in three groups of subjects: (1) famous saints or religious figures; (2) Protestant and Catholic clergymen enrolled in a year-long postgraduate course in pastoral care and counseling; and (3) hospitalized psychiatric patients. It is a clinical, in-depth study of a relatively small number of individuals. For the sake of brevity, I have had to condense a great amount of material and therefore must at times formulate impressions or opinions without presenting the data on which they are based. However, samples of both autobiographical material and interview data, as well as a description of the interview technique that is the main "research tool" I have used, are available in previously published studies [7, 8]. Further samples of these interviews, not elsewhere published, are also available in Pruyser's *A Dynamic Psychology of Religion* [5].* In the case of the

* The author gratefully acknowledges the assistance of his colleague, Paul Pruyser, Ph.D., for his careful reading and cogent suggestions on this chapter.

study of great religious figures and saints, it was necessary to resort to autobiographical reports. In my investigation I have made no efforts to define religion; rather, I haγe allowed my subjects to define their *own* religion as they were able to relate it.

EXTRINSIC AND INTRINSIC RELIGION

In attempting to break down such data into categories, some freshness and wholeness of the picture is lost, but there is a distinction between two types of religious sentiment, introduced by Gordon Allport [1], that I have found helpful in assessing religious practices and attitudes.

It was Allport's belief that much of what has been written about religion by Freud, as well as by many other psychologists and psychoanalysts, has to do with what he calls *extrinsic* religious attitudes, which are essentially utilitarian and used to meet narcissistic, defensive, or infantile purposes of the personality:

Extrinsic religion. For many people, religion is a dull habit, or a tribal investment to be used for occasional ceremony, for family convenience, or for personal comfort. It is something to *use,* but not to *live.* And it may be used in a variety of ways: to improve one's status, to bolster one's self-confidence, to enhance one's income, to win friends, power, or influence. It may be used as a defense against reality and, most importantly, to provide a super sanction for one's own formula for living. Such a sentiment assures me that God sees things my way, that my righteousness is identical with his. I see the nature of being as conforming to the facts of my particular being. Two pious, aged sisters were quarreling. One said with asperity to the other, "The trouble with you, Jane, is that you lack the grace of God in your heart." The grace of God, it seems, is hers, not Jane's.

By contrast, Allport describes *intrinsic* religion as follows:

. . . the intrinsic form of the religious sentiment regards faith as a supreme value in its own right. It is oriented toward a unification of being, takes seriously the commandment of brotherhood, and strives to transcend all self-centered needs. . . . a religious sentiment of this sort floods the whole life with motivation and meaning. Religion is no longer limited to single segments of self-interest. It is integral, covering everything in experience and everything beyond experience; it makes room for scientific fact and emotional fact. It is a hunger for, and a commitment to, an ideal unification of one's life, but always under a unifying conception of the nature of all existence.

The distinction between these two types of religious attitude will be developed further below. However, I take Allport's two types indeed only as types; in the actual lives of real people one will find ratios of intrinsic and extrinsic religion rather than simple intrinsicalness or extrinsicalness.

RELIGIOUS CONVERSION AND PSYCHOLOGICAL CHANGE

The process of religious conversion is of special interest to the psychiatrist because it seems to include elements of severe psychopathology. Like other acute psychological crises, it may or may not result in improved reality adaptation, but does usually result in some form of change or restructuring of the personality [9]. Most of the comments that follow are based on a detailed study of auto-biographical and biographical material of three great religious figures, Martin Luther, St. Augustine, and St. Ignatius of Loyola. I have reported on the first two in previous papers, so my present comments will focus primarily on St. Ignatius.

St. Ignatius lived in the sixteenth century and was a military leader before his conversion and subsequent founding of the Jesuit Order. During his convalescence from a severe leg wound suffered in a military engagement, he went through a long mental and religious struggle, questioning his past ways and yearning to find a religious vocation, in a sense substituting a religious identity for a military one. In the process of his struggle, during which he withdrew from contact with other people, fasted, and went for long periods without sleep, he had at least two experiences of illuminanation, during which he saw visions and subsequently experienced great relief from his suffering and obtained a "new" view of himself and the world. Despite the subjective similarity of these two conversion experiences at the peaks of their intensity, the subsequent results were quite different. After the first experience, notwithstanding an initial feeling of joy and release, there was a gradual deterioration with a severe depressive reaction in which Ignatius was tempted to suicide. It was only following the second and last experience that Ignatius' life changed significantly and in a constructive direction, so that he was able to gain the prodigious energy and inspiration to found and lead a new religious order.

The close relationship between religious conversion and acute mental illness is striking. In Ignatius' case, as in the conversions of many other great religious figures, the typical psychopathology of an acute depressive or psychotic episode is there. Why one may result in a "rebirth" into a better integrated life and the other in a crippled life is a difficult question to answer. Of course, these alternatives are available for any acute mental illness just as they are for any religious conversion. Conversion, like acute psychotic illness, must be understood as a *process,* not an event.

It is not accidental, I believe, that in all the religious crises I have been able to study that result in conversion and subsequent productivity and creativity, there is always a significant person available to listen or offer support occasionally. In Ignatius' case it was his confessor, who would listen patiently to Ignatius' highly emotional self-castigations and torments and then say, essentially, "Take it easy on the fasting, young man."

The role of regression seems to be a prominent factor in such conversions (in Ignatius' case the regression necessitated by his broken leg forced a passive, contemplative attitude upon an otherwise active man). Ignatius seemed to utilize this regression for resolution of conflicting intrapsychic elements. Essentially, this process involved giving up active male sexuality for what appeared temporarily to be a more regressive, passive dependence on God, but which actually resulted eventually in more mature and productive interpersonal relationships.

The relationship between religious commitment and identity formation, together with the important role of social factors in such changes in direction, has been amply discussed by Erikson [2]. I would like to focus on another dimension of the problem, which I do not think has received significant attention. The accounts of conversion experiences of these *homines religiosi* raise the question of normal and pathological narcissism. In my view, it is around this struggle that much of the conversion process seems to be taking place. After Ignatius' initial, "incomplete" conversion, there are strong megalomanic features. Despite all the talk of God, the saints, and piety in general, there was an expansive, self-centered grandiosity in Ignatius' utterances at the time. His plans for great pilgrimages seemed to have more to do with dreams of phallic conquests, outdoing the saints, and other exhibitionistic inclinations only faintly disguised behind a facade of being a special servant of God (more special than anyone else, in fact). Perhaps Ignatius himself sensed the falseness regarding his newly won "spirituality" at this point. At any rate, the egocentricity of his spiritual idealism became gradually transformed in an extremely painful, desperate, almost suicidal process, as one by one these vainglorious trappings were exposed and recognized for what they were. *This kind of transformation of narcissism is the essence of the process of conversion into an intrinsic religious orientation.*

It is this process that is so traumatic, *not* the turning away from worldly ambitions, sex, and so forth. For the latter can be associated with all kinds of grandiose fantasies of special favor with God and superiority over others. Parenthetically, we might add that Roman Catholics have long recognized the dangers of celibacy in this regard, namely, that it inclines the priest to the erroneous belief that his celibate life *itself* gives him some special divine favor.

To continue this phase of the religious conversion process, there is then a giving up by the person of the self-centered expectation of putting his personal dreams into action for God's (his own) glory. All of this comes crumbling down in what might be termed a *nadir* experience, in which the futility of projecting one's own megalomanic, infantile demands and expectations onto God is realized with a devastating insight. It is in this sense that the expression "dying to life" is really met, I think. One dies to this kind of narcissism. At this juncture, perhaps we can also speak of the true meaning of the term *humility*.

It is now possible for all of the cathexes that have gone into these mostly unconscious conflicts and narcissistic strivings (which in many ways may have been necessary, even useful, to the individual's previous defenses and to his usual involvement in the workaday world) to become available, freed for use in the "new" relationship with God, with others, and with one's new vocation. All of these are now integrated and moving in the same direction. Reality is now seen "as it is," without the narcissistic defenses against the sense of reality that previously protected one's self-regard at the expense of true perception of self and the world.

This new perspective is extremely difficult to describe in scientific terms, but the language used to express this transformation seems universal regardless of the culture, religious tradition, or environment of the person [4]. Individuals undergoing such a change speak of being "purged," of seeing things in their "true light"; they speak of "purity" and "simplicity," of a new "unity." They no longer see themselves as better than other men but essentially *like* other men. Thus, all men are seen as valuable in the light of what seems to be a change in basic values. As expressed in Ignatius' autobiographical document, "Creation is no longer a threat but a friend." For now he had become *a part of* the entire cosmic process. This change represented not an abandonment of narcissism, of course, but a change in its quality. Hypothetically, we might conceive of an integration of very early fusion experiences (primary narcissism), as well as early primitive introjects, into the personality. This process seems associated with a reduction of projections, prejudices, hates, and other distorted perceptions. Omnipotence is given up, "creatureliness" is realized, and with it a new perspective on God (in the religious person) and man as well as self.

I have expressed this process in a dramatized form, but I think some elements of this basic psychological pattern are far more common among men than is generally realized. Psychiatrically speaking, we are dealing here essentially with the problem of character change. It seems best to think of all such transformations as partial, as incomplete, and they may occur gradually and less dramatically than I have outlined.

Studies of the most outstanding saints and religious figures disclose a great deal of human foibles and psychopathology. No serious student of human nature, whether religious or agnostic, should be troubled by such findings. Unlike their apologists, the saints themselves were humble about their weaknesses. If anything, it should fill us with the greater wonder that, carrying the burden of such inner conflict, they were able to integrate it and to achieve so much in the world. Perusing the autobiographies of such religious figures as Pope John XXIII, St. Augustine, or St. Ignatius reminds us of the perhaps disturbing fact that the difference between ourselves and those "saints," as in the case of the difference between ourselves and those "sick people," who happen to be patients, is not as great as we might like to think.

THE MINISTER'S RELIGIOUS LIFE

Most of the views expressed in this section were drawn from interviews with 22 clergymen involved in a course of pastoral care and counseling at a prominent psychiatric institution. The subjects were all within the middle or upper socioeconomic class, well-educated, and theologically sophisticated, and were about four-fifths Protestant and one-fifth Roman Catholic. No Eastern religions, no fundamentalist Protestant sects, and no Rabbis were represented. The limited number of subjects and the socioeconomic class, as well as the rather narrow range of religious affiliations, need to be borne in mind in evaluating the findings reported here.

Despite the small number of subjects, there is a great deal of data on each of them. Not only was each interviewed for one and a half to two hours about his religious life, but there was extensive biographical and historical information on all of them, as well as an autobiography. The results of a full battery of psychological tests administered by a senior clinical psychologist were also available.

Method

The clergymen who participated in this study did so voluntarily with the understanding that they were participating in a research study of religious experience. In the interview I focused primarily on the more subjective aspects of their own religious development as they were able to report it. My technique was to conduct an essentially open-ended interview; anything resembling a questionnaire approach was avoided. I went into detail regarding "peaks," conversion experience, and the phenomenon of the "call" because of the obvious psychological significance of such events and because they "stood out."

Early Experiences of Religion

Without exception, all of the ministers interviewed had early and frequent exposure to various forms of religion, both in the home and in the church community. Religious teachings were generally introduced early in the latency period. Significantly, this is concurrent with the individual's struggle to overcome the Oedipus complex and at the time of the development of the superego. Earliest remembered religious experiences and practices invariably had to do with magical thinking and a rather primitive view of God. Only a minority of the subjects recalled early impressions of God as a benign, loving figure; the majority seemed to project punitive, admonishing features onto their image of God from whom they asked favor or forgiveness.

All but two of the ministers spontaneously mentioned struggles with guilt over masturbation at puberty and related these to their religious beliefs.

Religious "Crisis" During Adolescence

I obtained a great deal of material related to adolescents' religion, especially conversion experiences, the "call," and development of religious vocation. In adolescence it seems that conflicts stimulated by resurgence of instinctual forces, the reawakening of oedipal conflict, and its relation to identity crisis especially tend to dominate the scene in religious experience at the time. A frequent precipitating event for such a crisis was a loss, such as the death of a parent or the loss of a girlfriend.

About half the subjects had what I call an adolescent religious crisis. This was usually associated with a buildup of depression, confusion, anxiety, and prayer, leading up to a "conversion" and followed by a definite move in the direction of a religious vocation. The type of resolution of these crises and the effectiveness of the subsequent religious vocation seemed related to two main factors: (1) the presence or absence of some stable religious identifications from childhood, relatively free from serious superego pathology (implicit here, I believe, is a relatively good "ego strength"); and (2) the availability of a "therapeutic" relationship with another person, a friend, usually an older man and frequently a minister with whom the young person could talk (*never* the father). If both these factors were present, the chances were more favorable for a reintegration of the personality and a less superego-dominated religious faith, together with a marked increase in general efficiency, productivity, and quality of object relationships. (I would regard a poorly integrated primitive superego structure as a particular vocational hazard among the clergy.)

If their early religious identifications were very rigid or punitive or if there was a poorly developed superego structure, and when a helping person was not available, the religious crisis frequently led to a depressive reaction and in two cases to a subsequent brief psychosis requiring hospitalization. Interestingly, in the latter two cases, where more immediate integration was not possible and depression and even a psychotic state developed, the eventual prognosis was good. Transient psychosis in these cases may have prevented a premature structuring and settling of the personality at an immature, pathological level. In several other cases the religious crisis or conversion resulted only in a partial resolution of conflict and seemed to serve the primary function of reinforcing defenses at the expense of considerable personality restriction and impaired object relations. This latter group experienced their religious faith as "driving" them, and they did not have as much apparent freedom and spontaneity in their subsequent development in comparison with the rest of the group.

From this material I am inclined to conclude that the typical religious conversion occurring during late adolescence is a highly important psychological event, but hardly a reliable experience on which to base a vocational commitment. On the basis of this limited number of interviews, I would venture to say that the majority of adolescent conversions no more reflect potential for religious maturity in the intrinsic sense than infantile oedipal fantasies reflect mature heterosexual love.

It is interesting that only 2 of the 22 clergymen interviewed could be described as falling under the "once born" category described by William James, namely, those persons who seemed to have developed smoothly, without crisis and conflict, steadily toward a highly integrated religion and personality structure. In such persons, peaks and conversion experiences or acute struggles are absent. My impression is that their religious life had a lackluster quality and that they had a slight to moderate restriction in their personal relationships, but I would not be able to say that this would be generally true of all such "once born" persons.

Religious Maturity

Another impression based on these interviews is at this point only speculative, but could provide a testable hypothesis. It is that intrinsic religion, as defined by Allport [17], does not develop until the late twenties, thirties, or even the early forties. Even then it seems to be an uncommon development. What seems to be involved in the few cases in which it does occur is an integration of religious values within the personality, rather than religion being used to maintain defenses and satisfy infantile, dependent needs.

The struggle to develop intrinsic religious attitudes seems related to the problem of overcoming problems related to self-centeredness.

One of the best case examples for this view can be found in Dag Hammarskjold's *Markings.*

PSYCHIATRIC TREATMENT AND THE PATIENT'S RELIGIOUS LIFE

Whether a patient is in psychotherapy or hospital treatment, attempts at dealing with his religious beliefs can present problems. Some of these are due to the patient's conflicts about religion and some to attitudes of the psychiatrist. The question often comes up how religion should be dealt with in disturbed clergymen or other patients with strong religious beliefs who come into psychiatric treatment. Not infrequently, a patient about to begin psychotherapy may ask his psychiatrist whether the treatment will cause him to lose his religious beliefs. I think it is impossible to answer such a question at the onset of treatment, but one can make some general statements about this matter.

If a patient has a deep religious faith of the more intrinsic sort, he is no more likely to lose this than an artist is likely to lose his creativity by undergoing treatment. Kubie has written at length on this subject. Those aspects of the patient's religious beliefs that are neurotic and that serve defensive purposes are likely to be lost. Indeed, in successful treatment they should be mitigated. When treatment reaches its goal, excessive guilt feelings and shame about sin are likely to be modified, and there is a tendency for the superego aspects of the image of God to become less dominant. The same holds true for the magical and infantile aspects of one's view of God, which almost invariably will be decreased in the course of effective psychotherapy. Thus, we can say that if a patient's religion is primarily serving an extrinsic, utilitarian purpose in the interest of defense, maintenance of the status quo, or the satisfaction of primarily infantile needs, it is very well possible that in the course of successful treatment the individual will indeed lose his religion and may become agnostic. But when religion is associated with basically sound identifications and introjections, treatment will generally result in a more realistic orientation as far as religious outlook is concerned, and there may be an improvement in the relationship toward God and in other relationships as well. A few ministers whom I interviewed reported a deepening of their religious faith following psychoanalysis or psychotherapy. This seems to have resulted primarily from the analysis of an extremely pathological relationship with a parent.

If the type of treatment is psychoanalysis or expressive psychotherapy, and the patient professes to be devout, it is inevitable that the patient's religious attitudes will be subject to scrutiny in the course of treatment. My experience has been that with clergymen patients the therapist must be prepared to deal with core character problems in connection with religious belief. Thus, crucial character problems may be missed if the therapist himself steers clear of the patient's religion. For example, a 40-year-old Episcopal minister, who came into treatment following a depressive decompensation of his compulsive neurosis, prided himself on very proper attitudes toward his parishioners and his highly organized, regular participation in prayers and worship services. Only in the inflection of his voice and his facial and bodily mannerisms did the patient reveal a condescending contempt toward the therapist, toward his parishioners, and toward God and Christ. On one occasion, after several months of little change in treatment, the patient reported an incident in which he tossed his prayer book onto a table and had the intrusive thought, "What a bunch of crap." Further exploration of this disparaging attitude that the patient had unwittingly held both toward his God and in his human relationships resulted in a more productive turn in his psychotherapy and a significant improvement in his relationships.

The clergyman patient's resistance to having his religious beliefs examined is often due to strong aggressive or infantile wishes, but it is at times based on a striking emptiness in the religious life. Many clergymen who suffer from emotional difficulties serious enough to come into the psychiatric hospital have profound character pathology involving addictions, perversions, and behavior disturbances.

Such ministers, who are referred after serious trouble in their church or following some kind of scandal, may reveal, after careful examination, a long-standing paucity or complete absence of prayer life or any kind of feeling of closeness to or belief in God. Generally, this emptiness in the religious life parallels an impoverishment in all personal relationships. Religionists used to call this *acedia,* which was considered both suffering and a special sin.

In schizophrenic or borderline patients who give evidence of a fairly active religious life prior to decompensation, there may recur a strong interest in resuming religious activities after the acute disorganization begins to remit. Especially in very ill paranoid schizophrenic patients, religious interests may be connected with a delusional system. This may deter the psychiatrist from permitting the patient to participate in religious services, because such participation is viewed as "sick" and a continuation of the illness. A 20-year-old schizophrenic boy who had been hospitalized several times since the age of 13 developed a personal and bizarre variation of the Catholic faith and in the hospital expressed a strong desire to participate in Catholic services and to have time off for private devotions in his room. Such activities interfered to a certain extent with the time schedule of patient activities, so his psychiatrist objected. The patient became quite disturbed, but the psychiatrist, feeling his position was sound, was unrelenting. The impasse continued for several weeks as the patient gradually regressed and became acutely paranoid. Finally, following a change of physicians, the patient was permitted to participate in religious services under the firm guidance and structure of a priest. The patient was able to make a marginal adjustment, his acute psychosis went into remission, and he has been able to live outside of the hospital for many years subsequently. In retrospect, it is clear that this patient had managed to structure his entire life around religious devotions in the church, albeit in a rather peculiar and idiosyncratic way. For this man, religious practices served adaptive purposes, despite the fact that according to ordinary criteria the patient was living out what would be considered a psychopathological relationship to the Church and to God. The point is that for this highly obsessive man with a strong need for distance in interpersonal relationships, this was the most stable relationship he seemed capable of.

In my experience, psychiatrists 'occasionally miss potentials in their patients for using religion as a resource for improved adaptation. The problem is not that the psychiatrist needs to espouse religion in some way vis-à-vis his patients, but that he should not permit biases regarding religion to blind him to its possible use for his patient's rehabilitation.

General descriptions such as "religious" or "nonreligious" can be meaningless, and there is considerable difference of opinion among psychiatrists as to what constitutes religiosity in a patient. The most striking example of this is reported in a study in which all the staff psychiatrists of a private psychiatric hospital listed in two contrasting groups those patients whom they considered either actively religious or nonreligious. One hospital psychiatrist listed one of his patients as actively religious, and the same patient's psychoanalyst listed the patient in the nonreligious category! Both were senior staff members and both had been involved in the treatment of this patient for more than two years.

CONSIDERATIONS FOR FUTURE STUDY

Psychologically speaking, man's highest religious values can be viewed as existing on a continuum with psychopathology, not opposed to or separate from it. I hope the material presented on St. Ignatius has illustrated this point. For each of the human virtues frequently associated with religion (for example, self-sacrifice for others), there is a counterpart in psychopathology (for example, moral masochism). Psychoanalysis, with its insistence on calling attention to the falseness of much of what often passes for human altruism, sharpens our vision of true virtue and human love.

As William James stated in his classic, *The Varieties of Religious Experience*, people do not just have a God, they *use* their God. This has been the foundation stone of psychological studies of religion. In a recent report by the Group for the Advancement of

Psychiatry, "The Psychic Function of Religion in Mental Illness and Health," the authors outlined the psychic uses to which the human being puts a system of faith and worship [6]. This essentially functional approach to the psychology of religion has proved fruitful. Religious beliefs are indeed expressions of, and fulfillments of, man's oldest, most urgent wishes. Functional approaches do not solely comprise adaptive or defensive uses of religion. But in my view, the essence of religion also comprises *integration,* not just repression or need gratification.

In referring to Anton Boisen's *The Exploration of the Inner World,* Pruyser [5] stated:

. . . Boisen put a new stamp on psychopathology and religion by placing both in a framework of the life crisis. Mystical experience can best be understood if it is seen in the same order of intensity and depth that attaches to severe mental illness. Both are processes of disorganization and reorganization of personality, of transformation, dealing with man's potentialities and ultimate loyalties. I think that this is a position which places religious experience functionally and experientially most clearly at the nexus of holistic, integrating tendencies of the organism. In this theoretical framework, religion is not an adjuvant to integration; it *is* integration.

I believe this strikes very close to the core of the problem of the psychological exploration of religion.

In conclusion, I would like to make a plea for further exploration of what the late Gordon Allport referred to as intrinsic religious sentiments. In some of his last work, Allport was able to show that extrinsic religious attitudes were associated with high ethnic prejudice, and that intrinsic religious attitudes were associated with low ethnic prejudice. It is difficult to conceive of a more timely topic for research efforts, therefore, than further investigation of the relations between the intrinsic and extrinsic aspects of religious behavior.

The so-called intrinsic religious attitude is of course not necessarily related to any particular religious affiliation. But all of the great religions have much to say about the achievement of such a common goal, whether it be called "mystic selflessness," the polished personality of Zen, the intrinsic religious person, or the fully mature human being.

Man has split the atom, orbited in space, and probed the laws of the universe. Now a perhaps more formidable task awaits us: the exploration of our own inner nature, so that we can control our devisive tendencies and awaken the "still-slumbering affinity" that links us to our fellowman.

REFERENCES

1. Allport, G. W.   The religious context of prejudice. *J. Sci. Stud. Relig.* 5:447, 1966.
2. Erikson, E. H.   *Young Man Luther.* New York: W. W. Norton, 1962.
3. Freud, S.   From the History of an Infantile Neurosis. In *The Complete Psychological Works of Sigmund Freud* (Std. ed.). London: Hogarth Press, 1955, Vol. XVII.
4. Huxley, A.   *The Perennial Philosophy.* New York: Meridian Books, 1962.
5. Pruyser, P. W.   *A Dynamic Psychology of Religion.* New York: Harper & Row, 1968.
6. The psychic function of religion in mental illness and health. *Group Advance Psychiat.* [Rep.] 67, 1968.
7. Woollcott, P.   Creativity and religious experience in St. Augustine. *J. Sci. Stud. Relig.* 5:273, 1966.
8. Woollcott, P.   The psychiatric patient's religion. *J. Relig. Hlth.* 1:337, 1962.
9. Woollcott, P.   Erikson's Luther, a psychiatrist's view. *J. Sci. Stud. Relig.* 2:243, 1963.

The Role of Religion in Psychotherapy

E. MANSELL PATTISON

INTRODUCTION

Prior to World War II, literature on religion in psychotherapy was virtually nonexistent. Subsequently, the development of a rapprochement between psychiatry and religion has produced a large number of alliances between mental health professionals and clergymen. However, instead of clarifying past theoretical conflicts, these alliances have created marked confusion about the respective roles of psychotherapists dealing with religion and clergymen conducting psychotherapy [7, 11, 26]. A plethora of controversial literature has emerged, but the issues at hand have remained obscure.

In this chapter, I shall present an analysis of the differentiation of the social role of healer in contemporary society as it has emerged and differentiated over time. I shall suggest that as social roles of healing have differentiated, they have obscured basic differences in ideological position. These differences in ideological position may not necessarily be reconcilable at the present time. However, I shall suggest that many ideological problems may be resolved by closer attention to different forms and goals of psychotherapy. Thus, certain forms of psychotherapy may be enhanced by closer ties and involvement of religion in psychotherapy, whereas in other forms of psychotherapy this may be contraindicated.

ATTITUDES TOWARD RELIGION IN PSYCHOTHERAPY

Actually, little psychiatric discussion of religion has dealt with psychotherapy per se. More typically, psychiatric papers have dealt with theoretical analyses of religious behavior. Some work has appeared on the psychotherapy of religious persons, the diagnostic use of religion, or the importance of spiritual values [1, 2, 16, 19–22]. More recently, some authors have suggested religiously oriented psychotherapy [4, 5, 18, 28, 29]. However, most psychotherapists have tended to steer clear of dealing with religious issues in psychotherapy, much less employ religious concepts or techniques in their psychotherapy. Yet Ostow [23] has reported that as much as 40% of random selected psychoanalytic material may have religious connotations; Lowinger et al. [17] have demonstrated that the religious attitudes of psychotherapists significantly affect their treatment attitudes; another study [32] shows that religious roles affect psychological testing; and Szasz [31] reported the strong pro and con religious biases of a sample of psychoanalysts.

Klausner [11], a psychologist-sociologist, has recently suggested that professional attitudes toward religion in psychotherapy can be usefully analyzed by classifying attitudes according to task differentiation and role differentiation of the therapist.

Task Differentiation	Role Differentiation	
	One Role	Two Roles
One Task	Material reductionists	Alternativists
	Spiritual reductionists	
Two Tasks	Dualists	Specialists

The reductionists maintain that there is only one task and one role. The material reductionists claim that mental health is solely a question of scientific psychology, while the spiritual reductionists phrase the entire problem in religious terms. The dualists believe that there are both spiritual problems and psychological problems, but that one qualified person can accomplish both tasks. The alternativists claim that there is only one problem, usually psychological, but that either a minister or a psychotherapist can do the task. Specialists maintain that there are two tasks, one psychological and one spiritual, and that each task requires the respective specialist.

Historically, and in primitive societies, mental illness is a spiritual illness—a spiritual reductionism—and there is one role—that of the shaman, who is priest-therapist. In the most primitive societies, the shaman assumes his role because of what he is, while in a more complex society he assumes his role because of skills and knowledge. Correspondingly, illness comes to be defined as a personal problem within (psychological), rather than an impersonal judgment from without (spiritual punishment). Cures, then, are ascribed to the medicine and not to the supernatural power of the healer.

The process of differentiation progressed in society into the medical model of mental illness, which now separates medical and spiritual healers. This led to the development of the *spiritual reductionists*. This occurred in those religious groups in our society where secularization of society has resulted in social agencies' assuming responsibility for individual welfare, leaving the religious groups with few concrete contributions to individual or social welfare. In consequence, two antithetical theological attitudes developed. The fundamentalists rejected secular society and claimed that the only legitimate interest of the church was salvation in the hereafter, while some liberals moved toward a humanism that redefined salvation as solely the here-and-now welfare of man. The fundamentalists rejected psychology, while the liberals cloaked psychology in theology. So both groups became spiritual reductionists, although with exactly opposite goals, for the fundamentalists avoided psychology and the liberals sought to avoid theology.

The practical result is that the fundamentalist sects define mental health as a question of spiritual integrity to be treated by the spiritual methods of the minister, who is effective because of what he is, not what he does. A study at the University of Washington [9] found that fundamentalist ministers were defined by "spiritual call" rather than training, had the least education of all clergy, yet tried to handle the most counseling problems through spiritual methods alone. We can see that this task-role definition is much like that of the primitive shaman of the simplest society. That this can result in a successful practitioner is attested to by the success of the many faith healers.

On the other hand, in some liberal denominations the minister's task is defined as that of the psychotherapist, namely, the relief of psychological distress. The minister is effective because of what he does, not who he is, and is selected on the basis of training, not "call." He is a professional in direct competition with the secular psychotherapist, which he justifies by defining his task and role in religious terms. This movement is reflected by some pastoral counselors who do not work as clergy, but rather are in private practice as professional psychotherapists, declaring themselves to be "pastoral therapists."

The Chistian psychotherapists who reject the medical model are mostly *dualists*. They maintain that psychotherapy is but a prelude to spiritual therapy, which is the ultimate task of the therapist. They argue that psychosis is sin. The Viennese existentialists Daim [5] and Caruso [6] state that psychological problems reflect spiritual ones. Daim speaks of psychoanalysis as a "partial salvation" that introduces the patient to his need and treatment for "total salvation." Caruso says, "The object of all psychotherapy is . . . the acknowledgement of a transcendent hierarchy of values which should become, according to individual possibilities, a truth expressed in terms of one's own life . . . this existential synthesis, however, can be free and effective only if it results from . . . psychological analysis."

It should be noted that these men are not like the fundamentalists in disavowing psychology, but there is a similarity in that their psychology devolves upon Christian presuppositions—that psychotherapy is ultimately a religious task, and the role of the therapist is a spiritual one.

The medical specialist model is also rejected by a growing group of therapists influenced by the emphasis in medicine on the whole person, in psychology on holistic personality theories, and in psychotherapy on the existential aspects of human relations, which have fostered a therapeutic approach to the person in both his psychological and spiritual aspects. Generally couched in existential terms, this position maintains that the therapist must use both psychological and spiritual techniques to attain both psychological and spiritual goals. Some who advocate this position make no specific theological claims except generic moral ones; these include men like Frankl [6], many existentialists, and Rickel, editor of the *Journal of Psychotherapy as a Religious Process.*

In contrast to the spiritual reductionists and dualists, the *material reductionists* claim that there is but one task, and they deny the presence or relevance of spiritual aspects of man. In the past, some of these men, including Freud, felt that scientific psychology would replace the neurotic anachronisms of church and clergy. Today, however, most of these advocates accept religious activities as perhaps acceptable social means of achieving psychological goals. This *alternativist* position makes the clergyman the poor man's psychiatrist. The specialists see a collaborative relationship between psychological and spiritual, but no necessary integrative one.

As can be seen, the ideological position that a psychotherapist assumes may directly affect how he handles the religion of his patient, what religious concepts he may or may not introduce into psychotherapy, and how he may relate to the clergy and their work. In actual practice, however, these lines may be blurred, as will be illustrated in the next section.

PSYCHOLOGICAL AND SPIRITUAL GOALS IN PSYCHOTHERAPY

Here I shall suggest four different patterns of religious involvement in psychotherapy. I will assume a psychological-spiritual dichotomy, although the material would be explained by the material reductionists or spiritual reductionists solely within their own framework. I mean to illustrate, however, that much of the controversy over religion in psychotherapy depends on the frame of reference of the psychotherapist, and what transpires in therapy may depend not only on the actual behaviorial interaction, but also on the meaning ascribed to that behavior by both the therapist and the patient.

Psychological Means to Psychological Goals

Thirty years ago, Robert Knight [12] reported the psychoanalysis of a minister as an unusual event. Today, we have accumulated much experience in treating religious persons. The therapeutic process may result in drastic changes in a person's religion. He may give up his religion, which we must recall was considered necessary for successful therapy by some of the early psychoanalysts. More recently, a number of psychoanalysts have reported on the return to religion or strengthening and deepening of religion as the result of therapy. Linn and Schwarz [14] found 17 such cases, and Bowers [1] states that the task of the therapist is to reconcile the unconscious religious attitudes of the patient with his conscious theological attitudes. In these instances, psychotherapy contributes to spiritual goals, but only incidentally. The spiritual benefits are a consequence of the changes in the individual that make possible spiritual commitment and maturation.

It should be added that religion is often used as an ego-defensive maneuver. Ostow [23] reports that depressive patients often become religious as they become depressed, lose their religiosity as their depression deepens, become religious again as they improve, and give up religion when they recover. Novey [22] describes the use of religious institutions as a defense, and Stern [29] warns therapists about false spirituality that is a protective facade. For example, many fundamentalists would rather account for their problems as spiritual malaise instead of as a personal difficulty. Here again, psychological therapy may result in changes in the patient's perspective and use of his religion.

Clinical data indicate that religious groups may influence the development of character traits and that the religious person presents particular technical problems in the conduct of psychotherapy. Changes in religious commitment and behavior do occur as a result of therapy, which, depending on the nature of one's religion, may either be strengthened or discarded. In these instances, the therapeutic methods and goals are psychological, yet they do contribute to spiritual changes.

Psychological Means to Spiritual Goals

Men have three Gods: God as he is, God as my group sees him, and God as I see him. Freud was quite correct in *The Future of an Illusion* when he described God as the projected father figure. What others have since shown is that God is also a projected mother figure, or even a very primitive part-object from early infancy. Often a patient's reaction to God is based on these early childhood percepts, and his behavior reflects irrational early emotional object identifications rather than any rational, mature, theological concept of God. Consequently, how we experience God as a person may bear little relation to our verbalized theology of God.

Numerous authors have stressed the parallel between the patient-therapist relationship and the patient-God relationship. If the patient has disturbed experiences in the areas of faith, trust, and hope in his human relationships, he can hardly be expected to experience healthy faith, trust, and hope in relation to God. Bruder [3] emphasizes that the curative factor in therapy is relationship and that both sin and mental illness involve separation from God, one's neighbor, and oneself. Therapy at the psychological level provides the integration necessary to achieve synthesis at the spiritual level. As Smet [28] says, one must experience the basic elements of love, faith, trust, and hope at the human level before one can experience them with God. In this sense, then, the "corrective emotional experience" of psychotherapy may be a necessary prelude to healthy spiritual experiences with God.

The learning of religious *concepts* is quite different from religious *experience* when seen in this perspective. Take, for example, the child in relation to his parent. The child experiences his parent long before he has much conceptual appreciation of the child-parent relationship. Psychotherapy may clarify distortions of God, just as it clarifies distortions of the parents; however, this does not make the relationship with God or parent any more or less genuine. The therapeutic contribution is a clearer perception of the relationship that may enable the person to change his relationship to God.

In sum, psychotherapy can contribute to emotional experiences that the person may then use in his spiritual experiences, and it may clarify distortions of his relationship to God. It is important to emphasize that a "spiritual" psychotherapist is not necessary to accomplish these tasks, although a therapist who envisions these goals may be in a better position to turn the patient in these directions. Actually, a competent "secular" therapist may contribute more in this direction than a "spiritual" therapist who neither provides the necessary emotional relationship nor has the technical and personal skill to help clarify the patient's religious distortions.

Spiritual Means to Psychological Goals

Some current existential therapists argue that existential-spiritual conflicts may lead to psychological symptoms. Frankl [6] calls this "noogenic" neurosis. However one phrases it, the claim is that unless the existential-spiritual conflict is resolved, the psychological neurosis will remain. Caruso [4] puts it that a fundamental shift in values must occur before a person can adequately deal with his neurosis.

Less philosophically, Salzman [27] has described the maturational, integrative value that religious conversion may have in crystalizing a personality. Although all conversions are psychological phenomena at one level, and some conversions are solely ego-defensive maneuvers, a religious commitment and involvement may provide the necessary framework upon which psychological integrity can develop. Meehl [21] concludes that faith may assist in the mastery of neurosis, although it does not enable the person to overcome his neurosis. This is supported by published clinical reports on the integrative value of some religious experiences during the course of psychotherapy. In these instances, the psychological goals of therapy were assisted and implemented by the religious experience.

Spiritual Means to Spiritual Goals

The specialist would hold that the spiritual means of prayer, meditation, religious instruction, confession, Bible study, exhortation, and penance are the special province of the minister. In contrast, the dualist claims that the psychotherapist might well employ these techniques. At one extreme are those who argue that the therapist should ultimately transmit to the patient a philosophy of life. In specific Christian terms, Daim and Caruso argue that the therapist does not complete his task until he has brought the patient to a salvation experience. Others would not go so far in directly influencing the patient, although they would consider it appropriate to pray, meditate, share religious experiences, and offer explicit religious guidance. This may be because they feel that it will augment the psychological maneuvers, or they may wish to enhance the patient's spiritual life.

In each of these four instances, religion was a component part of the psychotherapy process. The degree to which it was so was dependent partially upon the religious attitude of the therapist and to a degree upon the religious attitude of the patient. It might well simplify matters to suggest that therapist and patient should have matching religious attitudes. However, that is impossible for the most part in a pluralistic society. Even more importantly, it ignores the question as to whether or in what circumstances it is therapeutically helpful or destructive to have religious congruence. I have here in mind the whole question of transference and countertransference aspects of psychotherapy in terms of religious issues— a matter untouched for the most part in psychotherapy literature [25].

A DIFFERENTIATION OF RELIGION
IN PSYCHOTHERAPY

At this point I wish to return to the issue of social differentiation of the healing role in society. In his book on primitive psychiatry, Kiev [10] has pointed out the importance of sociocultural context in psychotherapy. It is the sociocultural milieu that in large part determines the definition of mental illness, the nature of psychotherapy, who is patient, who is therapist, and what are to be the methods and goals of psychotherapy.

In primitive food-gathering societies, mental illness was social illness, because a necessary laborer was lost. Hence, treatment had a direct social rehabilitative focus. The shaman was effective because his role, methods, and social goals were accepted by him, by the patient, and by the society. The same is true for much of psychotherapy. If the goal is explicit social change, the therapist is quite directly the agent of his society—or a particular subculture of our pluralistic society.

If this is so, then in what way is contemporary psychotherapy any different from the primitive psychotherapy of the shaman? We can even go on to ask what psychotherapy means in our society, where it has come to include a friendly greeting, a few words of encouragement, or an inspirational devotional exercise. This loose thinking fails to differentiate between what is therapeutic and what is therapy. Both individual and group relations are "vital stuff" upon which our personalities feed in order to both grow and maintain ourselves as persons. Much of the criticism of psychotherapy has been based on the observation that no matter who does what to the patient, he gets better. Actually, this may only reflect the therapeutic, homeostatic, social milieu of the patient and the therapist. It is because he is a social agent that the shaman is effective in relieving symptoms and resolving intercurrent crises. It is at this level that much psychotherapy is conducted, although indications are that psychotherapy is probably not a very efficient method for either alleviating symptoms or resolving crises.

What scientific psychology and the development of a psychoanalytic psychotherapy have made possible are technical methods for effecting changes in the personality structure of the patient. In this situation, the patient and therapist still share common social values. They must even to make a therapeutic contract, but psychoanalytic psychotherapy is a special social activity whose purpose is to correct developmental personality distortions so that the patient will be better able to utilize the usual therapeutic social activities of life. Here therapy and therapeutic are complementary social interactions, although quite different in method and purpose. And in this instance the therapist is an agent of society, but only an indirect one, for the goals are primarily personal rather than social. So the goals of the shaman and the psychoanalytic psychotherapist are somewhat different.

This has implications for the techniques of psychotherapy. For the therapist whose goal is social change, it may be appropriate to employ social supports, as the shaman does. However, when the goal is personal change, it becomes important that the therapist remain apart from immediate social sanctions, that there be a social distance between patient and therapist, and that a nonnormative stance be taken by the therapist during therapy. Only when these conditions obtain can the therapy proceed toward its goals. Let us take an analogous example from child development. During adolescence the child commonly idealizes, imitates, and learns from his schoolteacher, who becomes a parent-surrogate. This nonhome parental figure is helpful precisely because there is a certain emotional and social distance between student and teacher. On the other hand the real parent is necessary to provide and maintain norms in the context of emotional-social closeness, which is necessary if the child is going to incorporate those norms into himself. The teacher and parent play complementary roles in accomplishing separate tasks, yet both are necessary if the child is to mature in normal fashion. In the same fashion, the psychoanalytic psychotherapist, like the teacher, is able to help the patient toward particular goals precisely because of his social-emotional distance.

What has occurred, then, is a differentiation of the shaman's priest-therapist role into two roles that are complementary. This differentiation does not imply that the therapist replaces the priest, nor that such differentiation is merely the result of secularization of society. The psychotherapist working toward social change may not actually be in a social role much differentiated from the shaman role. But for the psychotherapist working toward personal change, the technical demands require a sharp differentiation in the social situation [8].

If we examine the spiritual-psychological nature of psychotherapy in this light, we can see that the minister, like the parent, has a very close social-emotional tie with the patient and that this is an important advantage in his role as definer of social and moral values and behavior. It gives the minister as counselor a unique lever for dealing with certain social misbehavior and intercurrent life crises. Parsons [24] points out that, like a parent, the church is a necessary "boundary structure" for the maintenance of both the personality and society. On the other hand, this very strength is its weakness for the involvement precludes objective, detached analysis, as Szasz clearly indicates in his book *The Ethics of Psychoanalysis* [30].

In contrast, because of his social-emotional distance, the psychotherapist can challenge, explore, and clarify. But this very strength of psychotherapy is its weakness. Hartmann makes it clear that psychoanalysis provides knowledge but not guidance, that it makes for unity but not goodness, or as Ramzy says, psychoanalysis can only investigate values, it cannot create them.

Whether we take the parent-teacher model, or the minister-therapist model, we can see that each partner may ultimately have the same goal, which is the mature or moral child or patient. But either partner will fail if he attempts the task by himself. There is, indeed, a synthesis of goals, but the synthesis comes in the child or patient, not in one of the partners. If we now reconsider the question of spiritual and psychological goals raised previously, we can see that the minister-patient relationship precludes working toward some psychological goals, while the psychotherapist-patient relationship precludes working toward some spiritual goals. It is not that the goals are undesirable, but that the relationship is a limiting factor. This point is made clear by London in *The Modes and*

Morals in Psychotherapy [15], in which he observes that if we lived in a one-value society, the problems would only be technical ones. Since we do live and practice in a pluralistic society, it behooves the mental health community and the religious community to delimit more clearly the circumstances and patterns of use or management of religion in psychotherapy. The following recommendations may provide some guidelines for further investigation and clinical discussion.

1. It is the responsibility of the therapist to face openly his own ideological commitments in regard to religion in order to avoid countertransference biases and distortions. Countertransference problems may arise in treating both patients who share and patients who do not share the therapist's religious opinions.

2. For certain types of patients and for certain therapeutic goals, the utilization of religious concepts and practices may enhance the psychotherapeutic enterprise. This might occur most clearly in certain types of pastoral counseling. However, a mental health professional might employ religious dimensions in psychotherapy *if* there is *mutual* agreement between therapist and patient.

3. For certain patients and for certain therapeutic goals, as in the instance of characterological changes aimed at in psychoanalytic psychotherapy, *even if* the therapist and patient share religious views, it may be technically disadvantageous to introduce religious factors that might impede and interfere with the open exploration of the patient's characterological conflicts.

4. It would seem inappropriate in our pluralistic society to accept the claim of some dualists that the mental health professional has the privilege to attempt to change a patient's religion, i.e., to convert or deconvert a patient. In essence, without societal consensus, the therapist in a pluralistic society must place limits on his own personal goals and aspirations.

5. If we are to accept certain dualist propositions, represented primarily by some existentialists, that issues of meaning and value in life are indeed therapeutic concerns, then we must address ourselves as therapists to the appropriate technical maneuvers this may

entail and the appropriate safeguards that must be observed. Personally, I feel that there are merits in this existential position, but that we have not developed an adequate theory and method of psychotherapy in terms of this position. In my chapter on morality in this book, I have spelled out some preliminary concepts in this regard.

6. Finally, our discussion may imply that all psychotherapists are not in an ideal position to be of maximal value in psychotherapy to every patient. Every psychotherapist in a pluralistic society should be in a position to respond helpfully to all who seek help from him. Those in some type of public employ have an even greater responsibility. However, if we are to maximize the efficacy of psychotherapy, we may need to work toward a better matching of therapists and patients according to a number of variables, including the religious variable. Thus, if we can overcome our narcissistic needs as therapists, we may move toward greater interprofessional referral of patients to therapists who can be of maximal value to specific patients.

REFERENCES

1. Bowers, M. K. *Conflicts of the Clergy.* New York: T. Nelson, 1963.
2. Bronner, A. Psychotherapy with religious patients. *Amer. J. Psychother.* 18:475, 1964.
3. Bruder, E. E. Psychotherapy and some of its religious implications. *J. Past. Care* 6:28, 1952.
4. Caruso, I. A. *Existential Psychology.* New York: Herder & Herder, 1964.
5. Daim, W. *Depth Psychology and Salvation.* New York: F. Ungar, 1963.
6. Frankl, V. E. *Man's Search for Meaning: An Introduction to Logotherapy.* Boston: Beacon Press, 1959.
7. Franzblau, A. N. Distinctive functions of psychotherapy and pastoral counseling. *Arch. Gen. Psychiat.* (Chicago) 3:583, 1960.
8. Kadushin, C. Social distance between client and professional. *Amer. J. Sociol.* 67:517, 1962.

9. Kennedy, R. J., and Linsky, A. S. Attitudes and Activities of the Clergy in the Area of Mental Health. Unpublished manuscript, University of Washington, 1964.
10. Kiev, A. (Ed.) *Magic, Faith, and Healing.* New York: Free Press of Glencoe, 1964.
11. Klausner, S. Z. *Psychiatry and Religion: A Sociological Study of the New Alliance of Ministers and Psychiatrists.* New York: Free Press, 1964.
12. Knight, R. P. Practical and theoretical considerations in the analysis of a minister. *Psychoanal. Rev.* 24:350, 1937.
13. Lapsley, J. N., Jr. A Conceptualization of Health in Psychiatry. *Bull. Menninger Clin.* 26:161, 1962.
14. Linn, L., and Schwarz, L. W. *Psychiatry and Religious Experience.* New York: Random House, 1958.
15. London, P. *The Modes and Morals of Psychotherapy.* New York: Holt, 1964.
16. Lorand, S. Psychoanalytic therapy of religious devotees. *Int. J. Psychoanal.* 43:50, 1962.
17. Lowinger, P., Dobie, S., and Mood, D. Does the Race, Religion or Social Class of a Patient Affect His Treatment? In J. Masserman (Ed.), *Science and Psychoanalysis.* New York: Grune & Stratton, 1966, Vol. 9.
18. Mailloux, N., and Ancona, L. A Clinical Study of Religious Attitudes and a New Approach to Psychopathology. In H. P. David and J. O. Brengelman (Eds.), *Perspectives in Personality Research.* London: Crosby Lockwood, 1960.
19. Mann, J. Clinical and theoretical aspects of religious belief. *J. Amer. Psychoanal. Ass.* 12:160, 1964.
20. Mann, K. W. Religious factors and values in counseling: Their relationship to ego organization. *J. Counsel. Psychol.* 6:259, 1959.
21. Meehl, P. Some technical and axiological problems in therapeutic handling of religious and valuational material. *J. Counsel. Psychol.* 6:257, 1959.
22. Novey, S. Considerations on religion in relation to psychoanalysis and psychotherapy. *J. Nerv. Ment. Dis.* 130:315, 1960.
23. Ostow, M. Public address on religion in psychoanalysis, Cincinnati, 1964.
24. Parsons, T. Mental Illness and "Spiritual Malaise": The Role of the Psychiatrist and of the Minister of Religion. In H. Hofman (Ed.), *The Ministry and Mental Health.* New York: Association Press, 1960.

25. Pattison, E. M. Transference and countertransference in pastoral care. *J. Past. Care* 19:193, 1965.
26. Pattison, E. M. Social and psychological aspects of religion in psychotherapy. *J. Nerv. Ment. Dis.* 141:586, 1966.
27. Salzman, L. The psychology of religious and ideological conversion. *Psychiatry* 16:177, 1953.
28. Smet, W. Religious Experience in Client-Centered Therapy. In M. G. Arnold and J. A. Gasson (Eds.), *The Human Person.* New York: Ronald Press, 1954.
29. Stern, K. Some Spiritual Aspects of Psychotherapy. In F. J. Braceland (Ed.), *Faith, Reason, and Modern Psychiatry.* New York: P. J. Kenedy, 1955.
30. Szasz, T. S. *The Ethics of Psychoanalysis.* New York: Basic Books, 1965.
31. Szasz, T. S. The problem of privacy in training analysis. *Psychiatry* 25:195, 1962.
32. Walker, R. E., and Firetto, A. The clergyman as a variable in psychological testing. *J. Sci. Stud. Relig.* 4:234, 1965.

Morality, Guilt, and Forgiveness in Psychotherapy

E. MANSELL PATTISON

INTRODUCTION

Morality is an issue that has been debated but not systematically explored in much of the psychotherapy literature. At best, morality is generally viewed as irrelevant to psychotherapy; at worst, it is taken to imply a destructive antitherapeutic attitude. Yet in the face of these negative connotations there is a growing literature attesting to the centrality of aspects of morality to the psychotherapy enterprise [1, 12, 20, 36]. In fact, in my recent review [31] I have noted more than 160 recent entries in the literature on morality! In this chapter, I shall summarize a series of theoretical papers in which I have attempted to spell out a contemporary view of morality in psychiatry [24–31].

Past general attitudes about morality in psychotherapy may be summed up in four assumptions:

1. Morality was primarily the concern of cultural religion, which in turn was an oppressive force that inhibited rather than promoted human welfare.
2. Morality was an illusionary self-deception that prevented man from facing himself.

93

3. Morality was not a concern of psychotherapy, which was essentially an amoral scientific enterprise.
4. The psychotherapist played a nonmoral role, did not transmit his morality to the patient, and did not attempt to change the patient's morality.

In contrast, our data suggest the following assertions:

1. Morality is a central concern of society, not just the provincial concern of religion; and morality is primarily integrative rather than oppressive.
2. Although psychotherapy has exposed many misconceptions about morality, an adequate psychological theory of morality has yet to be developed. On the basis of contemporary ego psychology, I have proposed a concept of *ego morality*.
3. Rather than being amoral, psychotherapy has always been a moral enterprise, and morality has been the central issue of psychotherapy.
4. The psychotherapist *does* and *must* transmit his morality to the patient and influence the morality of his patient.

MORALITY AS CENTRAL TO SOCIETY

Freud's views on morality have been a cardinal influence in the thinking of psychotherapists. However, his writing dealt with such diverse aspects of morality that his ideas have been wrenched out of context or quoted without definition to such an extent that confusion rather than clarity has emerged. Freud did not elaborate a theoretical concept of morality, although certainly he was concerned with morality, as Philip Rieff argued in *Freud: The Mind of the Moralist* [33]. When Freud wrote specifically on morality, it was usually in regard to the psychopathologies of the superego. In *The Future of an Illusion, Civilization and Its Discontents,* and *Moses and Monotheism,* Freud identified morality with institutionalized religion; and both were ultimately related to superego development consequent to the resolution of the oedipal conflict. Thus, religion and its moral imperatives were an oppressive force that served to constrict man's freedom and foster illusionary denials of his basic nature and function. Freud's views on religion and morality were influenced by and consonant with the interpretations of anthropologists of his day. Freud noted that religion was not necessarily moral and had often been the source of oppression and destruction. This view is in part correct and needs little documentation. But this particular view of morality confuses morality with religion. Freud's critique of religious neuroticism has been taken to be a critique of morality. It fails to account for the normal and necessary functions of morality in the structure of personality, and it fails to recognize the central function of moral values in culture.

It is only because our contemporary American culture conceptualizes man as an individualistic organism that we can so conveniently overlook the cultural organizations that maintain our integrity as individuals. Our concern here is not with religion per se, but rather with religion as one mechanism that society has developed for codifying its morality. If we dispense with cultural religion as Freud recommended, we must still grapple with problems of developing an alternative social system of morality.

Clyde Kluckhohn [14] sums this up:

There is the need for a moral order. Human life is necessarily a moral life precisely because it is a social life, and in the case of the human animal the minimum requirements for predictability of social behavior that will insure some stability and continuity are not taken care of automatically by biologically inherited instincts, as is the case with the bees and the ants. Hence there must be generally accepted standards of conduct, and these values are more compelling if they are invested with divine authority and continually symbolized in rites that appeal to the senses.

No society can long function without a specific morality. Nor can this merely be left to individual discretion, for it is a group requirement as well.

Although it can be oppressive, morality is a central integrative force in culture. If religious faith is dispensed with, some other faith must replace it. In his important book *The Triumph of the Therapeutic: Uses of Faith after Freud* [34], sociologist Philip Rieff notes that psychoanalysis was instrumental in demolishing moralistic standards and rejecting religion. It thereby contributed to the symbolic impoverishment of our culture and to the establishment of "negative" communities that require no commitment and offer no integrative symbols. In the past, "positive" communities offered some sort of commitment and a type of salvation to the individual through participant membership. Rieff goes on to say:

> To speak of a moral culture would be redundant. Every culture has two main functions: (1) to organize the moral demands men make upon themselves into a system of symbols that make men intelligible and trustworthy to each other, thus rendering also the world intelligible and trustworthy; (2) to organize the expressive remissions by which men release themselves in some degree from the strain of conforming to the controlling symbolic, internalized variant readings of culture that constitute individual character. The process by which a culture changes at its profoundest levels may be traced in the shifting balance of controls and releases which constitute a system of moral demands.

In sum, morality cannot be ignored or dismissed, for morality, whether couched in religious institutions or not, provides a core integrative mechanism and content for the development of personality and for the maintenance of society. *Morality in these terms, then, is not a question of prohibitions, but rather of the values and definitions of appropriate behavior by which man governs his behavior.*

THE EGO IN MORALITY

In his recent review of theories of moral development, Nass [22] notes that psychoanalytic authors have at times distinguished between but at other times used interchangeably the terms *superego, ego ideal,* and *conscience.* Here, the superego, ego ideal, and narcissistic self will be considered in terms of their relationship to ego and the issue of morality.

Superego

In his 1914 paper "On Narcissism," Freud [9] anticipated a conceptual framework for morality: "It would not surprise us if we were to find a special psychical agency which performs the task of seeing that narcissistic satisfaction from the ego ideal is ensured and which, with this end in view, constantly watches the actual ego and measures it by that ideal . . . what we call our conscience has the required characteristics."

Here Freud intimated an *evaluative moral function of the ego,* which was to be further expanded into the concept of superego. This early broad concept of moral functions of the ego was to be narrowed as the superego concept was refined. The consequence was that in everyday clinical jargon we have since come to consider morality as solely a question of superego prohibitions.

But there is a distinction between unconsciously chosen moral values that are a function of the superego as a punitive condemnatory agency and consciously chosen moral values that are part of the conscious discriminatory ego. This distinction has not been made clear in psychoanalytic theories of morality, which have tended to focus only on the unconscious aspect of superego function. J. O. Chassell [2] has recently focused attention on the *variety of functions,* both conscious and unconscious, that are subsumed under the concept of superego: "The concept is most ambiguous, referring on the one hand to a narrowly delineated, specifically derived, separate agency of the mind 'determined by the earliest parental images,' and on the other to the complex process and structure implied in socialization."

Three general attitudes regarding superego morality have been taken. The first regards all superego morality as harmful and to be removed—one would be better off without much of a superego. This view, however, only considers the pathology of superego function.

A second view, represented best by O. H. Mowrer [21], recommends greater reliance on superego functions, based on the assumption that all guilt feelings refer to real moral violations. However,

Mowrer fails to recognize or accept the intrapsychic distortions that superego functions undergo.

The third view holds that superego function must be placed in appropriate balance. As an adult, one must realign one's superego according to one's adult ego value commitments, while modifying overly strict and erroneously developed superego sanctions. That is, one must learn not to feel guilty about inappropriate matters, and develop appropriate guilt for appropriate matters; appropriate guilt meaning a *signal of guilt,* rather than a punitive overwhelming condemnation.

This third view asserts that internalized superego norms, where appropriate and in the degree appropriate, serve as representatives of our group and cultural morals. Chein et al. [3] assert:

The social significance of the superego inheres precisely in the fact that it provides for individual standards of behavior not dependent on a person's limited experience and that their application is not dependent on the limited egocentric perspective of their situationally adaptive value to him. The social need of the superego type of morality rests, on the one hand, on the fact that the capacity of individuals to profit from experience or the range of individual experiences—even when vicariously augmented—are limited and, on the other hand, on the social necessity for a reasonably consistent set of standards even though the latter cannot be rigorously justified in experiential pragmatic terms.

In his *New Introductory Lectures,* Freud [10] comments along this line: "Fear of the superego should normally never cease, since in the form of *moral anxiety* it is indispensable in social relations, and only in the rarest cases can an individual become independent of human society." This collaboration of mature superego functions is highlighted by Edith Jacobson [13], who speaks of the development and modification of demanding, directive, prohibitive, and self-critical superego functions that become fused into collaboration with the ego. She comments: "Finally, the self-critical ego evaluates behavior not only in terms of correct or incorrect, true or false, appropriate or inappropriate, reasonable or unreasonable, but also from the standpoint of utilitarian or 'worldly' ego goals ('self-interests') with regard to their effectiveness and success . . .

the ultimate collaboration between self-critical superego and ego functions."

Ego Ideal

Various aspects of the affirming, loving, or approving counter-parts to prohibitive superego functions have been defined, apart from superego, as the ego ideal. In terms of morality, it is obvious that one's ego ideal plays an important role. However, the ego ideal may be modeled along destructive lines, for example, if one's ideal is John Dillinger. Or the goals may be too high, forcing the person to try neurotically and inappropriately to achieve those goals by fair means or foul. Or the ideals may be inappropriate to one's talent or role in life, as in the case of the intellectual but clumsy son of a ball player who cannot use his intellect because his internalized ideal involves physical prowess.

As with our analysis of superego, we cannot posit morality in terms of ego ideal alone. It provides powerful motivation and central values around which one's life behavior revolves. But unless the ego ideal is modified in alignment with reality and one's conscious value commitments, it may distort and pervert one's behavior, so that the end result is immoral rather than moral behavior.

The Narcissistic Self

A third intrapsychic source of morality involves the narcissistic self. One must accept, love, care for, and reward oneself before one can do so for others. Much pious self-abnegation and self-denial arises out of fear and anxiety about gratifying oneself directly; and so, vicariously and pseudoaltruistically, one gives to oneself through others. This is moral masochism—paying a price for one's pleasure by giving to oneself via others. Unfortunately, this is hostile giving and leads to the attempt to control and dominate others so that one will have foils through whom one can nourish the necessary narcissism of the self.

Kohut [16] sums up the role of the narcissistic needs of the personality and its ambitions as becoming "gradually integrated into the web of our ego as a healthy enjoyment of our own activities and successes and as an adaptably useful sense of disappointment tinged with anger and shame over our failures and shortcomings."

The person who has a grandiose image of himself, as well as the person who has a morbid self-image, will neurotically distort his behavior to balance the needs of the narcissistic self. These internal demands of ourselves must be aligned with our capacities and our conscious value commitments. If not, these internal self-needs will override whatever conscious moral compunctions one might have —a hungry man steals bread. On the other hand, the needs of the self, appropriately construed, provide a necessary balance between the commitment to self and the commitment to others that is *necessary for moral interpersonal relations.*

Ego Morality

Now we come to the role of the ego in morality. The contributions of the superego, ego ideal, and the narcissistic self are more or less unconscious, predetermined by our childhood experiences, and are in need of realignment in accord with the requirements of reality and the adult values to which one chooses to commit oneself.

Existentialists have long emphasized the role of personal freedom, responsibility, and decision in contrast to the unconscious, determined, irrational aspects of behavior emphasized by classic psychoanalytic formulations. In recent years, however, the ego psychologists, particularly Hartmann, Rapaport, and Erikson, have systematically elaborated the role of so-called autonomous ego functions. I have summarized this previously [26]:

Although couched in various terms, there is a growing consensus that personality development reflects not only physiological needs, but also value needs. Such needs to "make sense out of the world" have been termed the "quasi-needs" of the ego (von Bertalanffy), the will to meaning (Frankl), ego efficacy (White), and cognitive coherence (Festinger). Now, according to Hartmann's formulation of ego development, there is an initial undifferentiated id-ego

matrix from which emerges aspects of ego function separated apart
from instinctual drive processes; and these autonomous ego activities are involved in the process of developing a coherent effective
adaptation to the external world.

These autonomous ego functions assume the function of "ego
drives" in contradistinction to "instinctual drives." These ego
drives are dependent upon the beliefs and values of the culture
and these drives become important if indeed not the overriding
determinants of behavior. Thus it can be seen that belief systems
or value systems are the data that the ego uses to organize individual behavior. The lack of such cultural value data results in the
failure to develop an effective coherent ego structure; or the cultural value system may result in significant distortions in the formation of ego structure. Belief systems, whether they be religious
or otherwise, then are both necessary and influential in the development of personality.

The autonomous adult ego, then, chooses the values, morals,
norms, and standards by which the person shall live. These consciously chosen values, however, must be related to the unconscious
values of one's superego, ego ideal, and narcissistic self. The capacity to pursue moral behavior in adulthood optimally occurs
when there is a synchronous alignment between all four derivative
forces: superego, ego ideal, narcissistic self, and autonomous ego
values.

Morality has been usually thought of in terms of static rules, and
has been defined as a negative behavior related to avoidance of
punitive superego sanctions or meeting ego-ideal demands.

In contrast, the concept of morality developed here is a dynamic
concept emphasizing the selection of goals and values and the
process by which the person makes value choices; although including avoidance behavior, it emphasizes the positive goal-person-
directed behavior of the ego. This concept of ego morality posits
that there is an evaluating and coordinating structure and function
of the ego, which is part of its autonomous function, concerned
with defining and directing one's life in accord with the values one
has chosen.

This latter function of the ego is related to what Engel [6] calls
signal-scanning affect. His description of the nature and function

of this ego mechanism bears directly on our theoretical model of
ego morality:

> The *signal-scanning* affects have as their distinguishing character-
> istics a warning or signal function and a "how am I doing?" or
> scanning function, yielding information to self and to the environ-
> ment of good or bad, success or failure, pleasure or unpleasure.
> They serve as signals and means of reality testing for orientation to
> both external reality and internal reality "in a continuum extend-
> ing in all shadings from massive affect experience to mere signals
> and even signals of signals." (Rapaport) They have both *regulatory
> and motivational properties* . . . the signal-scanning affects operate
> to provide information which is then used by the self-inspection
> part of the ego as a guide for subsequent ego activities in the ser-
> vice of the reality principle.

The role of the ego in morality is also differentiated by Piaget [22]
in his studies on the development of moral concepts in childhood.
Early first morality is "moral realism," which is absolute and a
morality of constraint. This morality is superego moralism. The
child's morality is based on authority and fear of punishment.
Morality is a static set of absolute rules. In contrast, in adolescence
the child begins to develop a "morality of cooperation," which is a
relativistic concept. Morality here is related to ego functions of perception, evaluation, and determination of both consequences and
desires. It is a relativistic morality in that the adolescent learns to
guide his value choices and behavior in terms of his commitments
to others and to the ideals and goals he posits for himself.

Again, Chassell [2] notes that "children who were fixed in a state
of moral realism by their peculiarly strong ties to their parents were
unable to pass on to moral relativism, and remained bound by the
moral realism of the superego."

Recent studies on the development of moral character and moral
ideology have found that ego strength and "good moral character"
are closely associated. *It is ego strength rather than superego that
results in moral behavior.* Reviews [15] of child-rearing practices
reveal that parental attempts at specific training in "good" habits
fail to produce consistent moral behavior; whereas effective nur-

turance of a child as a significant, lovable individual with the use of firm, kind, consistent discipline does produce "moral capacity."

Ego morality I define, then, as the *process and mechanism* of balanced interdependent interplay between superego, ego ideal, narcissistic self-image, and autonomous ego values. Ego morality is the consequence of ego development, such that ego is the *final common pathway* for the establishment of values and moral choice to which the several forces of the personality have contributed.

The concept of ego morality implies that each individual is not alone in determining his value commitments and determining moral choices. The individual is molded by both his culture and his upbringing. His mature commitments are influenced by his social matrix, and his mature moral decisions are not his alone to make, but are interdependent on the judgments and evaluations of his peers. This is what theologians call "contextual" or "consensus" ethics.

Erikson [7] implies this interdependence in his discussion of the roots of virtue. He notes that man is not guided by a comprehensive and conclusive set of instincts, but must learn to develop what he calls the eight cardinal virtues of hope, will, purpose, skill, fidelity, love, care, and wisdom. He goes on:

The cog wheeling stages of childhood and adulthood are truly a system of generation and regeneration—for into this system flow and from this system emerge those attitudes which find permanent structure in the great *social institutions*. I have tentatively listed these social attitudes as reverent, judicious, moral, technical, ideological, interpersonal, productive, and philosophical. Thus the basic virtues—these miracles of everyday life—seem to provide a test for universal values, and to contain the promise of a possible morality which is self-corrective as it remains adaptive.

What Erikson intimates, and what ego morality posits, is that the individual optimally acts to integrate his behavior into the commitments to himself and to his society according to a whole range of social values. In some instances only a matter of personal preference is involved, while in others it is a question of decision for one's whole culture.

Guilt, Responsibility, and Forgiveness

From the central axiom of ego morality stem certain corollaries in regard to guilt, responsibility, and forgiveness that are of importance in terms of systematic theory as well as in practical application in psychotherapy [27, 29, 30].

I define four types of guilt: (1) civil objective guilt, (2) psychological subjective guilt feelings, (3) existential ego guilt, and (4) ontological guilt.

Civil guilt is arbitrary and impersonal. It is the violation of objective rules. Such guilt may or may not be related to morality. For example, the Jewish martyrs to Nazi justice were objectively guilty of violating Nazi law; or a small child may be objectively guilty of property damage. Many instances of civil guilt involve other types of guilt. However, objective civil guilt does not in itself indicate either the morality of the act or the moral consequences for the person.

Psychological guilt is an affect or guilt feeling. It is the subjective experience of internal condemnation of oneself by one's superego. Guilt feelings bear no necessary relationship to either existential ego guilt or civil objective guilt. To avoid confusion, I do not believe that the common word "conscience" should be used either for guilt feelings or for superego function, since these concepts refer to specific intrapsychic dynamics.

Existential ego guilt is a violation of relationship between man and man. This guilt, too, is objective, for it is a condition of estrangement between two persons. Existential ego guilt is ultimately a reflection of man's denial of his values and commitments, a denial of his true situation, and a withdrawal into narcissistic isolation from others. Existential ego guilt is not a feeling, but a situation.

Ontological guilt may be understood in theological terms as original sin, that is, man's basic responsibility for his life and behavior. In *The Brothers Karamazov*, Dostoevski puts it that man is responsible for everything and therefore guilty of everything. Sartre pessimistically notes that man can face only himself in making decisions; he has nowhere to turn to affirm that his decisions are right or moral. Ontological guilt is a reflection of the original state of man in the human condition of inadequacy: the fatal flaw of human character that leads man to damn himself; the classic theme of *hubris* of the Greek tragedians; the leitmotiv of our contemporary novelists, as in William Golding's *Lord of the Flies*; the basic contention of both ancient theology and the modern formulations of such theologians as Reinhold Niebuhr. Ontological guilt, in summary, is a situation, a reflection of man's awareness of what he is. One contemporary psychoanalyst, Allen Wheelis, in his metaphorical analysis of the limitations of self-enlightenment, *The Illusionless Man* [37], concludes that the ontological quest for meaning in life is crucial, yet unanswerable, and certainly untreatable by the psychotherapist.

The psychotherapist can and does address himself to the other three forms of guilt, however. Consequently, we must inquire into the management of guilt by the psychotherapist in terms of the concept of ego morality.

A typical therapeutic ploy has been to assume that behavior must be based on choice to be moral, and that one should not feel guilty about one's behavior that has been unconsciously determined. The assumption here is that guilt and morality are integral to each other. However, this view does not account for the variety of circumstances that we call guilt. Indeed, psychotherapists have for the most part concerned themselves with reducing guilt feelings, but they have ignored the "existential guilt situation."

In contrast, I propose that morality is only tangentially related to guilt feelings and is primarily involved with existential guilt— that is, the issue of relating to others in terms of one's ego commitments to them.

Out of existential human incapacity rises the conflict between one's own conscious aspirations and one's own unconsciously determined behavior. Indeed, St. Paul's classic self-confession states: "I do not do the good things that I want to do, but I do practice the evil things that I do not want to do."*

* Romans 7:19, Williams translation.

It seems fatuous to assume that by rational process we can analyze our behavior into determined and chosen components, as
Farber [8] points out. One's moral choices are a *combination* of
conscious and unconscious motives and norms, and a combination
of determined and free choices. I suggest that we never know fully,
in any conscious rational sense, what our motives are or why we
choose the way we do. The concept of a rational man is at best a
partial truth—the only people that seriously attempt to live by
reason alone are paranoids! I assert that we need to rely upon and
utilize in an integrated fashion our unconscious and irrational aspects of self as well as our conscious and rational self.

Furthermore, I submit that we are often faced with situations
in which we cannot determine either beforehand or afterwards
whether the alternative we chose was more moral than the other.
In Sartre's analysis, we often cannot look to arbitrary external
norms, or to others, or to a scientific analysis. Rather, we must accept the fact that existential choice is made by us. That alone may
on occasion define our choice as moral. *I have chosen with integrity
and that makes it moral.* In terms of psychotherapy, Lewy [19] concludes: "A person must be able to take the consequences of and be
willing and able to answer for what he thinks, feels, or does; to
acknowledge and feel that this is a part of himself." Ego morality
implies that one makes one's choices with as much integrity as one
has and accepts the consequences of those choices with the same
integrity.

We are responsible for everything we are and do. But responsibility does not imply that we should be punished even if guilty, in
the sense of blamable. Superego moralism condemns the self as
worthless and bad, whereas ego morality appraises the self with integrity without either rejecting or punishing it. Superego moralism
says, "I feel guilty"; whereas ego morality says, "*I am guilty.*"

The task of the psychotherapist, then, is not to assuage guilt feelings, although that is often a necessary preamble to successful
therapy. Rather, the therapist seeks to help the patient to see himself and his relationships with others in the light of how the patient
violates the relationships to which he is committed. The resolution

of guilt feelings does not change the basic violation of relationship, which is existential guilt. Patients would quite willingly settle for pacification of their superego, but they are reluctant to undergo the pain of changing their pattern of relationship so that they no longer need to feel guilty!

This, then, leads to the problem of forgiveness. Psychological guilt feelings can be resolved by appeasement, restitution, paying back, or making up. Here, punishment is the price one pays to the superego to stop making one feel guilty. This is what I call the punitive model of forgiveness, which is not forgiveness at all. But one must learn to stop punishing oneself, for it is of no value to anyone. Rather, one needs to face up to one's existential guilt. As a result, this sense of guilt may be more deep, for one must stop making pretenses and acknowledge oneself for what one is. Only when one has come to grips with the sort of person that one is can one hope to be a responsible, moral person, rather than merely to evade or placate one's superego. Punishment is no solution to the problem of existential guilt, for it is the hostile, defiant, rejecting *attitude* toward authority, one's own integrity, and one's true being. Here it is learning to accept oneself when one realizes that one is unacceptable; and seeking reconciliation from the estrangement one's behavior has brought. This is what I call the reconciliation model of forgiveness [27].

In terms of ego morality, the question is not one of guilt feelings, but rather of the assessment of what one is and how one behaves in order that one may modify one's behavior in terms of one's conscious moral commitments. Guilt feelings are of value as signal affects that the ego must then assess as to their validity and use as spur to action. The resolution of a situation in life in which one has violated one's moral commitments is not via punishment but rather via reconciliation.

PSYCHOTHERAPY AS A MORAL ENTERPRISE

It has been popular to assert that psychotherapy is not concerned with morality because psychotherapy is a scientific enterprise. However, as we are all aware today, this issue of morality in science looms large. More importantly, psychotherapy is a social enterprise and thereby comes under normative social sanctions [20, 23]. Note that psychotherapists would not long be in business if our society did not approve of us and support us!

The psychotherapist cannot escape from the issues of morality by pleading neutrality. There is a degree of neutrality, but that is different from noninvolvement in morality. Thus, Ginsburg [11] states: "There is no escape for the therapist from the problem of values which indeed become his basic concern permeating all his therapeutic efforts." What makes issues moral in psychotherapy is that they affect the life and welfare of human beings. To assume that the task of psychotherapy is merely to make the unconscious conscious and that it makes no difference how the ego decides is fallacious. Lewy [19] comments that it cannot be assumed that the analyst keeps hands off morality, for the therapeutic goal is to help the person to assume moral responsibility. The therapeutic task is not only to provide the patient with the freedom from neurotic conflict, but also to provide him with the freedom to become a moral person.

Levi-Strauss [18], the anthropologist, indicates remarkable parallels between the primitive shaman and the psychoanalyst. In both instances, there is a "belief consensus" between the patient, healer, and audience. The shaman was effective because his role, his methods, and social goals were defined by his society and accepted by him and the patient. The same is no less true today of psychotherapy. If the goal is explicit social change, the therapist is quite directly the agent of his society, as, for example, the prison psychiatrist who attempts to rehabilitate the criminal. In everyday psychotherapy with psychotics, children, and adolescents, most of us use direct, explicit, value-laden techniques. As a matter of fact, *most* of our usual psychotherapy is much more aimed at social change and based on social norms than we would like to believe. We are able to do this because society has defined it as appropriate, and our middle-class therapist-patient-society system is so congruent that we fail to see the social mandate under which we operate.

(This assumption is rudely brought to our attention, however, by the difficulty in conducting therapy with patients of either higher or lower social strata, much less patients of non-American cultures.) This is not necessarily bad. As a matter of fact, it is inescapably necessary when the goal is social change.

It is because he is a social agent that the shaman is effective in relieving symptoms and resolving intercurrent crises in the life of his patients. The psychotherapist, too, is a social agent. But scientific psychology and the development of a psychoanalytic psychotherapy have provided a technical method for changing the personality in addition to just social rehabilitation. Yet in this situation, the patient and therapist still share common social values. They must even to make a therapeutic contract. Although psychotherapy is a special social activity with an immediate goal solely related to the patient, the ultimate goal is that the patient will be better able to return to society. Here the therapist is an agent of the society, but only an indirect one, since the goals are immediately personal rather than directly social.

Where the therapist is a direct agent of the society, his role as a definer of values is more obvious. However, I suggest that even in the most autonomous psychoanalysis, the analyst is nonetheless the agent of the society. On the other hand, the therapist is an agent of the patient in all instances, and this makes the psychotherapy relationship different from educational or social enterprises and persuasion techniques, *for the goal of the therapist is to enhance the patient's capacities to deal with his society rather than merely to make the patient conform to society.*

The task of the therapist, then, is to help the patient achieve the capacity to live a moral life according to the society of which both are a part. The society "hires" the therapist in a sociological sense to restore one of its members to function, while at the same time the therapist is not a direct agent of the society, but rather the direct agent of the patient. This serves as a corrective and protection against the inevitable constrictions of society, for by developing the capacity for ego morality the therapist frees the patient from the unconscious irrational hold of society on the patient. Further, the patient is now free to participate in constructively changing his society. By this fact, *the therapist indirectly is himself an agent of change in the society of which he is a part.* This function may be ultimately his most important contribution to society. For like the artist, poet, and scientist, the therapist is a member of the "mediatorial elite," who are the agents of change so necessary to alleviate the constrictions of society. Hence, in the terms of Philip Rieff's analysis [34], the patient who develops an adequate ego morality can utilize the integrative and maintaining symbolic values that are necessary for the maintenance of himself and his society; but he also has the capacity to serve as remissive agent in challenging accepted values in a constructive and creative way.

In summary, to say that morality is a central concern of psychotherapy means that psychotherapy is ultimately aimed at clarifying the values to which the patient is committed, defining the values by which the patient wishes to pattern his life, and enabling the patient to synchronize his actual behavior with his goals and values. Obviously, this is a far cry from reinforcing without inquiry the patient's value system, "moralizing" by either patient or therapist, or perpetuating the "moralisms" built into the neurotic structure of the patient's life.

It may be that as a consequence of therapy the patient will continue to maintain many of his prior life values. But now the patient holds his life values for perhaps different, mature reasons rather than on the basis of anachronistic neurotic needs.

THE TRANSMISSION OF MORALITY IN PSYCHOTHERAPY

The assertion that psychotherapy, especially psychoanalysis, is an ethically neutral and value-free interaction has gone by the board in the light of numerous studies that demonstrate that therapy is most successful when there is value-congruence between therapist and patient, and, more importantly, that the therapist does, indeed, transmit his values to the patient. In recent reviews, Ehrlich and

Weiner [5] and Krasner [17] conclude that the experimental evidence is overwhelming on the transmission of values. That is no longer debatable. The issues now are (1) how this influences therapy; (2) what the values are that a therapist holds and transmits; and (3) how the therapist influences the values of his patient.

The more directive therapies are neither more nor less desirable because they are more directly value-bound and directly aimed at specific social behavioral changes. The real problem lies in situations in which the patient-therapist-society consensus *does not obtain*. Let me describe three different situations of belief consensus, ranging from very specific values, actions, and goals to nonspecific values, actions, and goals.

1. A specific religious community may request psychotherapy for members of its community. Here the therapist must at least be sympathetic to the values and goals of the religious community if he is to fulfill his obligation to both the individual and his community. An example might be a therapist working at a religious college.
2. A social institution may request psychotherapy for a person under its jurisdiction. An example might be a therapist in a prison or a children's home.
3. A society may provide general social support and sanctions for a person to seek psychotherapy. An example would be a psychotherapist in private practice.

In these three examples, there is a consensus in each instance. In the first, there is a very specific value system and very specific goals. The therapist is committed *in the therapy* toward transmitting and working toward specific values. As a consequence, the goals of therapy are limited, the freedom of the patient is limited, and the degree of patient change is limited. In the second instance, the values and goals are less specific, but yet there are constraints in terms of specific goals and the degree to which the patient has the freedom to choose them. In the third instance, there are no specific goals, and the values are those of the society at large. Here the therapist transmits the least specific values, and therapy is least aimed at specific changes in behavior. Rather, the goal is to achieve the *capacity* for commitment and choice within the general range of the society at large. This is the development of ego morality in its largest sense.

It is this last sort of therapy that Ramzy [32] describes as value-investigating, not value-creating. Or, as Hartmann [12] notes, psychoanalysis can make for unity but not goodness; psychoanalysis can enable us to understand how we create our values and enable us to act with integrity, but it cannot choose our values or establish the criteria that we shall use.

The psychotherapy relationship is not just another social relationship—it is a special and unique dyad. In psychotherapy, the social relationship is an "as if" situation that allows particular interpersonal interaction to develop for the purpose of therapeutic analysis. It is in the "as if" of the therapy that the psychotherapist sets aside any valuative or moral considerations. However, the "as if" nonmoral context can only be meaningful if it is ultimately related to the moral context and value concerns of the larger social context within which the psychotherapeutic "as if" relationship occurs.

As Tarachow [35] notes, the various models of psychotherapy can be described in terms of the degree of "as if" that obtains in the therapy relationship. The more bound to the external social context the psychotherapy model is, the more directly the values of the therapist and patient are involved. The more "as if" the therapy, as in psychoanalysis, the less directly the values of each are involved. But Tarachow points out that even so, the therapist's task is to relate the knowledge gained through the "as if" situation to the reality context of the therapist's and patient's world.

At this point it is clear that in developing a position on morality in psychotherapy, we must specify the model of psychotherapy, which ranges all the way from "social engineering" to Szasz's "autonomous psychoanalysis." In this regard, Cumming and Harrington [4] have demonstrated that "social distance" varies between therapist and patient depending upon the nature of the therapeutic contract, the social context of the therapy, and the social role of the therapist.

I propose, then, a general statement: *The more specific the value consensus of the patient-therapist-society, the more specific are the values transmitted in therapy, the more limited are the goals that can be achieved in therapy, and the more limited is the degree of change that is possible for the patient.*

From this general proposition, I suggest that the therapist has the obligation (1) to be aware of his own values; (2) to be aware of his patient's values; (3) to define the patient-therapist-society consensus within which he is working, and if he cannot work within that consensus with integrity, to refuse to treat the patient and refer the patient to a therapist who is able to work within that consensus; and (4) to maintain respect for the patient's integrity so that the patient is able to develop a distinction between the values of the therapist and the patient *even though they may be in agreement.*

Again, the problem is not that we transmit values, but rather what our values are and how we transmit them. The concept of ego morality implies that we do not wish the patient to change his values on the basis of unconscious and irrational forces, but rather on the basis of his own conscious ego values. It rejects the notion of the patient assuming values because he is dependent, because he is helpless, or on the basis of the transference in the therapeutic relationship.

Finally, the less specific the moral values the therapist transmits, the more opportunity the therapist has for helping the person to achieve the *capacity for ego morality.*

REFERENCES

1. Beres, D. Psychoanalytic notes on the history of morality. *J. Amer. Psychoanal. Ass.* 13:3, 1965.
2. Chassell, J. O. Old Wine in New Bottles: Superego as a Structuring of Roles. In R. W. Gibson (Ed.), *Crosscurrents in Psychiatry and Psychoanalysis.* Philadelphia: Lippincott, 1967.

3. Chein, I., Gerard, D. L., Lee, R. S., Rosenfeld, E. *The Road to H.* New York: Basic Books, 1964.
4. Cumming, E., and Harrington. C. Clergymen as counselors. *Amer. J. Sociol.* 69:234, 1963.
5. Ehrlich, D., and Wiener, D. N. The measurement of values in psychotherapeutic settings. *J. Gen. Psychol.* 64:359, 1961.
6. Engel, G. L. Towards a Classification of Affects. In P. H. Knapp (Ed.), *Expression of the Emotions in Man.* New York: International Universities Press, 1963.
7. Erikson, E. H. The Roots of Virtue. In J. Huxley (Ed.), *The Humanist Frame.* New York: Harper, 1960.
8. Farber, L. H. *The Ways of the Will.* New York: W. W. Norton, 1963.
9. Freud, S. On Narcissism. (1914). In *The Complete Psychological Works of Sigmund Freud* (Std. ed.). London: Hogarth Press, 1955, Vol. XV.
10. Freud, S. *New Introductory Lectures.* New York: W. W. Norton, 1933.
11. Ginsburg, S. W. Values and the psychiatrist. *Amer. J. Orthopsychiat.* 20:466, 1950.
12. Hartmann, H. *Psychoanalysis and Moral Values.* New York: International Universities Press, 1964.
13. Jacobson, E. *The Self and the Object World.* New York: International Universities Press, 1964.
14. Kluckhohn, C. Introduction. In W. A. Lessa and E. Z. Vogt (Eds.), *Reader in Comparative Religion: An Anthropological Approach.* New York: Harper & Row, 1966.
15. Kohlberg, L. Development of Moral Character and Moral Ideology. In M. L. Hoffmann and L. W. Hoffman (Eds.), *Review of Child Development Research.* New York: Russell Sage Foundation, 1964, Vol. 1.
16. Kohut, H. Forms and transformations of narcissism. *J. Amer. Psychoanal. Ass.* 14:253, 1966.
17. Krasner, L. Behavior Control and Social Responsibility. In A. P. Goldstein and S. J. Dean (Eds.), *The Investigation of Psychotherapy.* New York: Wiley, 1966.
18. Levi-Strauss, C. The Sorcerer and His Magic. In *Structural Anthropology.* New York: Basic Books, 1963.
19. Lewy, E. Responsibility, free-will, and ego psychology. *Int. J. Psychoanal.* 42:260, 1961.
20. Margolis, J. *Psychotherapy and Morality: A Study of Two Concepts.* New York: Random House, 1966.

21. Mowrer, O. H. *The New Group Therapy.* Princeton, N.J.: Van Nostrand, 1964.
22. Nass, M. L. The superego and moral development in the theories of Freud and Piaget. *Psychoanal. Stud. Child* 15:51, 1966.
23. Nelson, B. The psychoanalyst as mediator and double agent —an introductory survey. *Psychoanal. Rev.* 52:45, 1965.
24. Pattison, E. M. Social and psychological aspects of religion in psychotherapy. *J. Nerv. Ment. Dis.* 141:586, 1965.
25. Pattison, E. M. Contemporary views of man in psychology. *J. Relig. Hlth.* 4:354, 1965.
26. Pattison, E. M. The Effects of a Religious Culture's Values on Personality Psychodynamics. Read to Section H–Anthropology, American Association for the Advancement of Science, Berkeley, Calif., 1965.
27. Pattison, E. M. On the failure to forgive or to be forgiven. *Amer. J. Psychother.* 19:106, 1965.
28. Pattison, E. M. Toward a psychological theory of morality. *J. Amer. Sci. Affil.* 19:65, 1965.
29. Pattison, E. M. Morality and the treatment of the character disorders. *J. Relig. Hlth.* 4:290, 1967.
30. Pattison, E. M., Bishop, L. A., and Linsky, A. S. Changes in public attitudes on narcotic addiction. *Amer. J. Psychiat.* 125:160, 1968.
31. Pattison, E. M. Ego morality: An emerging psychotherapeutic concept. *Psychoanal. Rev.* 52:187, 1968.
32. Ramzy, I. The place of values in psychoanalysis. *Int. J. Psychoanal.* 46:97, 1965.
33. Rieff, P. *Freud: The Mind of the Moralist.* New York: Viking, 1959.
34. Rieff, P. *The Triumph of the Therapeutic: Uses of Faith After Freud.* New York: Harper & Row, 1966.
35. Tarachow, S. *An Introduction to Psychotherapy.* New York: International Universities Press, 1964.
36. Weisman, A. D. *The Existential Core of Psychoanalysis: Reality Testing and Responsibility.* Boston: Little, Brown, 1965.
37. Wheelis, A. *The Illusionless Man.* New York: W. W. Norton, 1966.

PART II
CLINICAL STUDIES OF RELIGIOUS
BEHAVIOR

This section deals with the clinical interpretation of religious behavior. At the clinical level, the therapist is faced with both the diagnostic assessment of religious behavior in patients and the treatment of symptoms related to religious behavior. At a theoretical level, we are faced with the development of scientific means of investigation and explanation of religious behavior, as well as the necessity of dealing with that perennial problem of normal versus abnormal.

Kiev provides a broad overview of these issues. Although he deals primarily with primitive religion, the principles he spells out are applicable to the more usual religious behavior encountered by the American clinician. Pattison and Casey present an in-depth study of glossolalia, a currently popular and controversial practice. Their data demonstrate the necessity for marshaling careful experimental and clinical data before drawing either theological or psychological conclusions. Pahnke applies experimental methods to mystical and psychedelic experiences. In addition to giving substantive results, he illustrates the use of experimental methods to elucidate religious conceptual issues. Mora provides a historical and clinical review of a familiar religious clinical syndrome—scrupulosity. In addition to describing its psychodynamics, he offers guidelines to treatment. Finally, Salzman takes up the study of religious conversion from a psychodynamic viewpoint. He extends earlier studies by looking not at the phenomena but at the person, showing that conversion may be either a maturational experience or a regressive pathological experience.

These chapters provide apt examples of the value both experimental and clinical research can bring to a balanced appraisal of religious behavior. Further, they emphasize that the study of religious behavior must be based on both the personal meaning and the sociocultural context of such behavior.

Primitive Religious Rites and Behavior: Clinical Considerations

ARI KIEV

INTRODUCTION

Primitive religion traditionally has referred to the specific beliefs and practices of aboriginal people, which according to Radin [22] pertain to "a belief in spirits outside of man, conceived of as more powerful than man and as controlling all those elements in life upon which he lays most stress." In this chapter, the concept of primitive is used in a broader sense to include contemporary religious groups whose activities have much in common with pre-literate religious practices—in particular, an emphasis on altered states of consciousness and other phenomena associated with the concrete manifestations of the spirit world.

A relationship between religion and altered states of consciousness has been recorded since ancient times. The ancient Greeks paid special respect to the oracle who could enter a trance. Divinely inspired seizures, trances, and visions were commonplace in biblical times. Glossolalia and dissociative states, which were associated with the Wesleyan revival in eighteenth-century England and with nineteenth-century American revivalist sects, have remained a major element in Fundamentalist religions to the present. The ethnological literature contains numerous accounts of ecstatic mental states in a wide range of cultures [7, 19, 20]. Unusual mental conditions such as hallucinations, hysterical seizures, and trance states played an essential role in religion in various cultures. Repeated illness, hysterical fits, and trance behavior are prerequisite experience for priests in a number of North American Indian as well as African and Asiatic tribes. Various techniques such as group rituals, breathing exercises, dancing, torture, and fasting, and various psychopharmacologically active agents such as alcohol, Indian hemp, peyote, and mescaline are often employed to induce unusual mental states for their presumed religious value and significance [16, 23].

The existence of sects and special groups that emphasize the development of unusual mental states is not restricted to underdeveloped societies. This has been shown in recent times in the various messianic sects of the more deprived socioeconomic and racial groups in the United States and in various nativistic movements among societies recently in contact with Western civilization, such as the peyote cult and the ghost dance religion of the North American Indians and the cargo cult of Malaysia [11, 24]. A considerable literature describes the function of such phenomena in supporting both the structure of institutions and the individuals within the society. Besides fulfilling religious needs by symbolically expressing customs and social relationships, rituals and beliefs have been viewed as supporting the individual participants while reinforcing the values of the group.

Religious sects offer answers to ultimate questions and goals that are more readily obtainable than those of the everyday materialist world. The possibility of self-improvement through participation is held out to all. To the extent that these groups are small, they can provide a sense of exclusiveness and a feeling of belonging to the community in which the individual is considered most important. These sociological and anthropological views emphasizing the integrative functions of religion have been supplemented in recent years by interest in the mental health potentialities of religious activities, many of which are clearly designated as healing procedures [5, 12, 13, 17, 18].

These issues were examined in *Magic, Faith, and Healing* [12], an anthology of primitive folk psychiatries, which focused on certain common elements in diverse psychological treatment approaches and on the relevance of specific cultural factors to both the content and technique of psychotherapy. One of its major inferences was that many primitive psychiatries are substantively psychological, even though they are methodologically unscientific and supernaturalistic. However, irrespective of the supernaturalist or magical methodology of primitive psychiatry, certain therapeutic factors were found to be operating in these primitive psychiatries that, on closer examination, were found also to operate in contemporary scientific psychiatries. These considerations suggested that the substantive psychology and the faith of the native healer in his system might be as important for successful treatment as the scientific accuracy of his methods. In particular, these studies underlined the emotional aspects of the therapeutic process, the nonspecific effects of therapy, the role of group forces, the powerful influence of the therapist, and the effects of cultural factors in a great range of primitive psychiatric treatments found throughout the world.

As in Western psychotherapy, it was found that in most instances the patient's favorable expectations were reinforced by the treatment setting and techniques and by the healer's faith in the patient's capacity to respond to treatment. At times, the healer's initial pessimism introduced ambiguity into the situation and increased the suggestibility and anxiety of the patient, promoting his desire to please the healer.

The connection of treatment with dominant values, by enlisting the valuable support of the community, further reinforced the patient's faith in the healer or healing society and his expectation of relief.

Suggestibility was often increased by participation in emotion-arousing group dances and songs, which further inclined patients to expect help. Community support, participation in healing cults, direct commands, reassurance, and environmental manipulation all were seen as realistic supportive elements that in themselves were anxiety-reducing.

Possession experiences, which were encouraged in certain healing cults, and group participation provide a number of additional therapeutic benefits, such as the attainment of high status through cult roles, the opportunity for acting out aggressive and sexual behaviors, the opportunity for reversal of sexual roles, and a temporary freedom from responsibility for actions.

Psychological defenses were also strengthened by readily available belief systems by which personal idiosyncratic difficulties could be explained in terms meaningful to the group and by opportunities provided for the active expression of aggression and other pent-up feelings. Thus, analysis of institutionalized witchcraft practices that also channel aggressive drives revealed that such benefits as psychological catharsis and social control could arise from what might even be illegal and antisocial practices.

In most of the societies examined in *Magic, Faith, and Healing,* the healer utilized popular notions of his own prestige and influence. These beliefs, coupled with his special techniques, were seen as permitting him to avoid intense emotional involvements with his patients. He received institutional support for the "objective" and neutral behavior, which not only reinforced the patient's trust in the treatment, but also minimized fears of his motives. By adhering to a standard social role, the healer gained the power of the role regardless of his personal qualities or abilities.

These studies of primitive psychiatries reveal the presence of certain factors not ordinarily emphasizd in examinations of the therapeutic elements of psychological treatments. In all the societies studied, treatment procedures were governed by particular rules, and the relationships among the healer, the patient, and the group followed prescribed patterns. One of the principal conclusions suggested by these studies was that these basic features of psychological treatment were as important as the features that differentiated them. The healers in all instances could bring a tremendous amount of personal influence to and arouse a multitude of emotions in the patient, as well as in the group, during the healing situation. This use of influence to arouse emotion was seen to have therapeutic value. In addition, the healer's ability in most instances to use the beliefs and ideas of the group as a fulcrum for influencing successful treatment led to the reintegration of the patient into the community.

Although such comparative studies are relatively new, recognition of the value of religious healing is not. Janet [9] devoted much of his writing to describing the therapeutic effects of such forms of healing as existed at Lourdes. Freud [6] in 1904 noted that the majority of primitive and ancient religious therapies must be classed under psychotherapy, for "in order to effect a cure a condition of 'expectant faith' was induced in sick persons, the same condition which answers a similar purpose for us today." In a detailed discussion of brief psychotherapy Fenichel [4] wrote: "The healing power of Lourdes or of a Catholic confession is still of much higher order than that of the average psychotherapist for neurotics are always more or less looking out for passive-dependent protection, for a 'magic helper.' The more a psychotherapist succeeds in giving the impression of having magic powers, of still being the representative of God as the priest doctors once were, the more he meets the longing of his patients for magic help."

THE FUNCTION AND SIGNIFICANCE OF PARTICIPATION

Religious groups such as snake-handling cults, American Indian peyote cults, and Pentecostal sects provide a form of social integration for individuals in anomic, stressful, and changing situations. They appeal to emotionally isolated groups in urban societies because they provide universal themes, structured world views, methods of attaining grace, contact with divinity, relief of distress, and salvation—the achievement of which are not dependent on special qualities, but only on faith and adherence to the group's tenets. In an achievement-oriented society, this is important for those without skills, resources, or the benefits of inherited social status.

Most of these groups provide social acceptance for everyone and

socially acceptable ways for releasing suppressed emotions and
frustrations. Being able to express oneself in a dramatic pantomime
or through the gift of tongues or in various very elementary dance
and song exercises enables the inarticulate to express themselves in
a stereotyped way in the presence of sympathetic participants. When
the conceptual focus is on the presence of evil and hopelessness in
the world at large, as it is in many Pentecostal groups, the group
offers the individual an opportunity to transfer his hopes to a
greater life in the hereafter. The material qualities of the larger
society, such as education, income, membership in the predominant ethnic and racial group, are minimized or on occasion viewed
as sinful. Faith and opportunities in the hereafter are emphasized.
The religious status that comes from participation is substituted
for socioeconomic and racial status and serves to integrate the individual into the group.

This is the function and the meaning of participation in these
groups. The regressive or dissociative phenomena that distinguish
these groups provide a dramatic vehicle for self-expression and
catharsis, which attests to the individual's faith and affirms the
validity of the group's beliefs, since the regressive phenomena are
taken as manifestations of a particular deity or spirit of the group.
To achieve even some degree of disinhibition does not require
intellectual skills, and even the lowliest person may be possessed
by the god.

It is important to note that regressive and dissociative practices
such as tongues, hallucinatory states, and trances are central to
religious rites in authoritarian or structured groups. During the
daily routine of their lives, the members are expected to attend
other meetings and informal social situations during which constraint is exercised over them.

THE PROBLEMS OF NORMAL AND ABNORMAL

Knowledge of primitive religious rites and behavior is of importance to the practicing psychiatrist who may encounter such

phenomena as glossolalia, faith healing, spirit possession, and drug-induced hallucinatory states in his clinical work with American Indians, Mexican-Americans, and other impoverished groups, as well as middle-class devotees of LSD and Eastern religions.

The psychiatrist may have difficulty distinguishing culturally acceptable behavior and ideas from the autistic behavior and thoughts of members of unfamiliar subcultures. Individuals have occasionally been diagnosed and treated for subscribing to beliefs that were misinterpreted and delusional. To avoid this, the psychiatrist must examine the beliefs of nonpatients from the same culture.

In an investigation of delusions of West Indian schizophrenic patients in England, I observed a predominance of religious and magical themes that were related to the beliefs of West Indians who valued a Fundamentalist view of the Bible, accepted the phenomenon of charismatic personalities and notions of *obeah,* ghosts, and religious healing [14]. There were, however, distinct differences in the use of cultural beliefs and practices by the normal and psychotic groups. The patients often distorted beliefs in idiosyncratic ways, outside the context of church services. West Indians who received a "call" and were moved to preach or establish missions were generally well integrated in other areas of their lives, unlike those patients who claimed to receive a "call" but who showed marked impairment in their lives. Possession by a "holy spirit," which leads to a "spiritual quickening" and ends in a sense of peace and relaxation, is a transient experience commonly encountered in religious services among West Indian Pentecostalists. In general, these experiences did not lead to overactivity or loss of conscious control over the expression of such feelings. The patients, however, could not maintain sufficient control of autistic and regressive behavior to be able to fit into the prescribed ritual pattern, and they expressed cultural notions in idiosyncratic ways that accounted for the differences between their delusions and the normal West Indian's beliefs. The schizophrenic patients were rarely humbled by such experiences and tended to overpersonalize and distort the significance of the biblical message in their unsuccessful restrictive efforts to explain their psychological or psychotic experiences. According to other West Indians, those who only claimed to be "called" could be distinguished from those genuinely receiving the "holy spirit," the experience of which could be witnessed.

Delusions, in contrast to beliefs, are generally over-inclusive, and the patient's life is so disorganized that diagnosis is not difficult. Where delusions closely parallel beliefs, emphasis must be placed on the relationship of the delusional ideas to the inner insecurities and morbid experiences of the patient. Thus, beliefs about *obeah*, black magic, evil eye, and other such notions might be considered as pathological or delusional when, as Cameron [3] has suggested, they "introduce behavioral distortion or impoverishment" and if they make a person "ineffectual in his social relationships or interfere with his attainment of important satisfactions." In addition, one must look for exaggerations, misinterpretations, and distortions of culturally acceptable beliefs; this ultimately necessitates either familiarity with the culture or consultation with representative members.

The diagnosis of psychiatric disturbance cannot be based on social behavior. It must be based on examination of the mental state. Deciding on what constitutes psychopathology when studying people from other cultures or subcultures is most difficult and has led to the view that illness or abnormality can be operationally defined rather than judged against an absolute standard insofar as the patient's symptoms can be viewed as either distressing to him or to the group. According to this view, it is not the idea but the way in which the idea is used by the individual and the nature of this use and distortion of belief relative to the standards of the group that are the crucial determinants of a psychopathological label.

SPIRIT POSSESSION

Spirit possession is a phenomenon known to mankind since biblical times. It refers to a relationship existing between spirits and humans manifested by the possession of the human being by the spirit, so that the behavior of the human is taken as the behavior of the spirit [21].

The induction of trance or possession states by various techniques is perhaps the most common element in primitive religious practices. It is also the most dramatic element of primitive religious practices and the most visble manifestation of the particular religious groups.

The quality of possession varies from one individual to another. Some enter possession states with relative ease through prayers and symbolic offerings. This usually applies to healers, mediums, and leaders. Save for the changed voice, posture, and facies, most preserve keen awareness of the ongoing situation and their role in it.

The possession states of others are often marked by a greater loss of self-control and consciousness. The range of spirits is so great that a large number of patterns of behavior appear acceptable as spirit possessions, which accounts for the recognition of the possession in nonparticipants and nonbelievers, a phenomenon that usually strengthens the belief of the believers.

The psychiatrist may at times be called upon to determine whether a patient experiencing a genuine religious ecstasy or possession state outside the ritualistic context is in fact suffering from psychiatric disorders of the hypomanic, manic, or schizophrenic variety. The distinctive characteristics of an ecstatic state are its transiency, ineffability, pleasantness, and noetic quality, in which new significance is found in the familiar. The individual may experience an absolute analgesia, a sense of calmness and inner peace, a sense of passivity, a feeling that the familiar has special significance [1, 2, 8, 10].

FOLK SYNDROMES

Occasionally, a psychiatrist may encounter patients who attribute their symptoms to such folk syndromes as bewitchment (*embrujamiento*), fright (*susto*), sorcery (*obeah*), angry spirits, or the evil eye (*mal ojo*) [12]. The first inclination is to think in terms of schizophrenic delusion formation. It should be emphasized, however, that belief in witches, for example, is not in and of itself pathognomonic of schizophrenia or any psychiatric disorder. Diagnosis must be based on the presence of such primary symptoms as loosening of association, a disorder of affect, ambivalence, and autism. A diagnosis of paranoid schizophrenia obviously creates more difficulty and requires scrutiny of ways in which the patient may distort culturally acceptable notions.

Treatment for such folk syndromes may be difficult and may require recourse to a representative of the particular subculture, who is usually equipped to reduce the culturally induced anxiety associated with special beliefs. Frequently, a patient in the early stages of a schizophrenic illness attempts to rationalize his difficulties on the basis of ideas derived from and acceptable to his group. This is an important point, since participation in such religious sects and cults frequently leads to a reduction in distress and a marked feeling of calmness. Religious groups usually offer explanations for many of the psychological changes patients may be experiencing. For this reason, participation may have an ameliorative effect on the course of illness.

PSYCHONOXIOUS PROCESSES

While many workers have pointed to the psychosocial benefits afforded by religious activity and participation in nativistic movements such as the peyote cult and the ghost dance religion of the North American Indians and the cargo cults of Melanesia, as well as in various Pentecostalist and Spiritualist sects, there is some evidence that participation may have an adverse effect on some individuals. The ill effects of revivalist conversion procedures were recognized by the New England preacher Jonathan Edwards, who, according to Sargant [23], made a practice of reducing guilt and acute apprehension as the first step towards conversion until the sinner broke down and indicated complete submission to the will of God. In instances of individuals already suffering from religious melancholia, the possibility of suicide or insanity was always recognized and was usually "put down to the debit side of the conversion ledger."

Study of Subud sects in England provided some clinical evidence that participation in religious activities promoting dissociative experiences could have deleterious effects [15]. The same thing holds for the dissociative experiences associated with LSD and peyote, in which the individual is so disoriented by the experience that his confidence in himself and his habitual ways of doing things is undermined and he becomes extremely dependent on present cues. This is fine if the individual is reasonably stable and there is a leader or a healer present who can utilize the regressive experience to help the person integrate his experience. The various perceptual and cognitive distortions that occur under the influence of the drug or under the influence of the group atmosphere require explanations, and if the individual cannot find an explanation for these experiences, he may explain them in terms of himself and be unable to differentiate himself objectively from the internal experience of distress. In this sense, the experience may be very undermining.

CONCLUSIONS

On the basis of this brief examination of some of the key issues in the study of primitive religious behavior and rites, one may conclude that participation per se in primitive religious rituals derives from a variety of motives and that it may have many beneficial effects in terms of growth of the individual, both from the point of view of the functions, activities, or involvement in the religious group and from the adoption of a rationale or philosophy or theology of life. Participation in and of itself is not pathological, nor is it harmful, although one must always remember that dissociative experiences may be very difficult for certain kinds of patients to tolerate. In summary, it is probably most helpful for neurotic patients, for those in borderline states, and perhaps for patients who are suffering from chronic schizophrenic illnesses and who therefore benefit from the integration into group activities in which they are able to participate. It is probably not as beneficial for people with acute psychotic illnesses and certainly is most dangerous when such participation is engaged in by people with acute organic illnesses, when the fundamental illness is not recognized by members of the group.

REFERENCES

1. Anderson, E. W.   A clinical study of states of ecstasy occurring in affective disorders. *J. Neurol. Psychiat.* 1:80, 1938.
2. Bleuler, E.   *Textbook of Psychiatry.* London: Macmillan, 1924.
3. Cameron, N.   *The Psychology of Behavior Disorders.* Boston: Houghton Mifflin, 1947.
4. Fenichel, O.   *Brief Psychotherapy* (Collected Papers, 2d series). London: Routledge, & Kegan Paul, 1955.
5. Frank, J. D.   *Persuasion and Healing.* Baltimore: Johns Hopkins Press, 1961.
6. Freud, S.   On Psychotherapy (1904). In *The Complete Psychological Works of Sigmund Freud* (Std. ed.). London: Hogarth Press, 1966, Vol. I.
7. Gee, D.   *The Pentecostal Movement.* London: Elim Press, 1945.
8. James, W.   *The Varieties of Religious Experience.* New York: Longmans, Green, 1902.
9. Janet, P.   *Principles of Psychotherapy.* Translated by H. M. and E. R. Guthrie. London: George Allen & Unwin, 1925.
10. Janet, P.   *De L'Angoisse a L'Extase.* Paris: Librairie Felix Alcan, 1928.
11. Kiev, A.   Psychotherapeutic aspects of pentecostal sects among West Indian immigrants into England. *Brit. J. Sociol.* 15:129, 1964.
12. Kiev, A. (Ed.).   *Magic, Faith, and Healing: Studies in Primitive Psychiatry Today.* New York: Free Press, 1964.
13. Kiev, A.   *Curanderismo: Mexican-American Folk Psychiatry.* New York: Free Press, 1968.
14. Kiev, A.   Beliefs and delusions of West Indian immigrants to London. *Brit. J. Psychiat.* 109:356, 1963.

15. Kiev, A. Subud and mental illness. *Amer. J. Psychother.* 18:66, 1964.
16. La Barre, W. Primitive psychotherapy in native American cultures: Peyotism and confession. *J. Abnorm. Soc. Psychol.* 42:294, 1947.
17. La Barre, W. Confession as Cathartic Therapy in American Indian Tribes. In A. Kiev (Ed.), *Magic, Faith, and Healing: Studies in Primitive Psychiatry Today.* New York: Free Press, 1964.
18. La Barre, W. *They Shall Take Up Serpents: Psychology of the Southern Snake-Handling Cult.* Minneapolis: University of Minnesota Press, 1956.
19. Lowie, R. H. *Primitive Religion.* New York: Boni & Liveright, 1924.
20. Norbeck, E. *Religion in Primitive Society.* New York: Harper, 1961.
21. Oesterreich, T. K. *Possession.* Translated by D. Ibberson. New York: Richard S. Smith, 1930.
22. Radin, P. *Primitive Religion.* New York: Viking Press, 1937.
23. Sargant, W. *Battle For The Mind.* London: Heinemann, 1957.
24. Wallace, A. F. C. The Institutionalization of Cathartic and Control Strategies in Iroquois Religious Psychotherapy. In M. K. Opler (Ed.). *Culture and Mental Health.* New York: Macmillan, 1959.

Glossolalia: A Contemporary Mystical Experience

E. MANSELL PATTISON AND

ROBERT L. CASEY

INTRODUCTION

As we move from the office to the community, psychiatrists and other mental health professionals encounter unusual behavior patterns, often in a religious context, upon which they are asked to submit professional judgment. The problems of interpretation have been highlighted by the recent work in psychiatric anthropology [1, 2, 7, 16]. However, the case of glossolalia presents an interesting problem closer to home—one on which mental health professionals have been consulted and their conclusions questioned. In this chapter, we shall briefly review this phenomenon as a case study in the interpretation of religious phenomena.

Glossolalia, or speaking in tongues, typically occurs in a small church or a small group of people. A member will suddenly burst out in unintelligible speech that sounds like gibberish. This is said to be the Holy Spirit speaking; and frequently another member will then "interpret" the message sent from God. The model for this experience is taken from the "Pentecost experience" recorded in Acts 2:1–4: "And when the day of Pentecost was fully come, they were all with one accord in one place. And suddenly there came a sound from heaven as of a rushing mighty wind, and it filled all the house where they were sitting. . . . and they were all filled with the Holy Ghost, and began to speak with other tongues, as the Spirit gave them utterance."

HISTORY OF GLOSSOLALIA IN WESTERN RELIGION

The Christian tradition of speaking in tongues antedates the New Testament Apostles. Glossolalia had been practiced for many years along with other ecstatic phenomena by the prophets of the ancient religions of the Near East. Prophets and mystics of Assyria, Egypt, and Greece reportedly spoke in foreign tongues during states of ecstasy and uttered unintelligible phrases said to be revelations from the gods. The Hebrew prophets appear to have similarly engaged in ecstatic states and practiced glossolalia. So the practice was not unknown, in all probability, to the early Christian Apostles [4].

In common with the religious scene today, there was ardent disagreement about the meaning of glossolalia among the early Christians. The onlooking crowd at the Pentecost experience thought the group of disciples drunk, whereas the Apostle Peter asserted that they had been speaking a new language. In subsequent debate during the next two centuries, five different positions on glossolalia were taken by various Christians: (1) that the spirit of God was speaking through the person, i.e., God possession; (2) that the devil was speaking through the person, i.e., demon possession; (3) that the person was given the supernatural ability to speak in a natural language; (4) that the person was given the supernatural ability to speak in a supernatural language; and (5) that the person was speaking in an oracular or cryptic manner that was a particular manifestation of a spiritual state.

Although the Apostle Paul warned against the enthusiastic excesses of first-century glossolalists, the issue remained unresolved. But it came to a head over the practices and spiritual claims of second-century followers of Montanus. Church councils then officially proscribed the practice of glossolalia. From then on until the sixteenth century glossolalia appeared sporadically, often associated with episodes of trances, hysterical states, and automatisms. In his classic history, R. A. Knox [11] describes all such phenomena as types of "ecstatic" or "enthusiastic" behavior. During medieval times this was almost invariably taken to be evidence of demon possession.

With the advent of the pietistic revivals of the seventeenth and eighteenth centuries, a new interpretation took hold. Dissatisfied with the intellectual rational concepts of religion, the pietists looked for direct human evidence for the existence and activity of God. Thus, seizures, trances, automatistic behavior, and glossolalia were now taken to be manifestations of possession by God. Small sects sprang up that practiced a wide variety of such "enthusiastic" behavior. Huguenot children in seventeenth-century France prophesied and allegedly spoke in unknown dialects. In the eighteenth century, Quakers and Methodists practiced glossolalia, and the nineteenth century saw the Irvingite movement in England.

In America, the "enthusiastic" movement spawned the Shakers. Glossolalia was practiced by the early Mormons, and a variety of indigenous sects took up and perpetuated glossolalia, along with other more dramatic activities such as snake handling, fire eating, poison swallowing, and faith healing [12, 19]. Around 1900 came the beginning of the Pentecostal movement, which became a major religious movement and now is one of the most rapidly growing religious groups in America.

In reviewing these "enthusiastic" groups, one notes a lack of uniformity of practice. Some sects practiced a whole gamut of trance states, automatisms, and hysterical symptomatology, while other sects practiced only one specific form of "enthusiasm," such as the quivering of the Shakers or the glossolalia of the Irvingites. Likewise, glossolalia may be associated with full-scale trance states or may be practiced by individuals during states of full consciousness with no other manifest changes in mien or behavior.

In the United States today, glossolalia is practiced by more than two million people. Among the lower social classes, particularly in the primitive remote regions of the South, glossolalia is only part of a full range of snake handling, convulsionary, hysterical behavior. But what has attracted interest in the past ten years is

the practice of glossolalia by members of the staid mainline denominations such as the Episcopalians, Lutherans, and Presbyterians.
Among urban middle- and upper-class churches, glossolalia is practiced as an isolated phenomenon by physicians, college professors,
captains of industry, even psychologists, who sit in full composure
and dignity while speaking in tongues!

GLOSSOLALIA IN NON-WESTERN SOCIETIES

Enthusiastic, ecstatic, mystic possession, trance states, and other
kindred phenomena have long been of interest to anthropologists
[8, 9, 16]. Glossolalia was known in ancient India and China, and
ethnographies describe glossolalia in almost every area of the world.
May [15] concludes:

As a rule, speaking-in-tongues and kindred phenomena are confined
to those areas where there is spirit possession and where inspirational shamans hold forth. Glossolalia can be and often is the
result of spirit-induced ecstasy making it possible for the inspirational shaman to cure, exorcize, and prophesy . . . speaking-in-
tongues is widespread and very ancient. Indeed, it is probable that
as long as man has had divination, curing, sorcery, and propitia-
tion of spirits, he has had glossolalia.

As with Christian glossolalia, primitive societies practice glossolalia
in a variety of forms and ascribe a variety of meanings to it. In
some societies it is a concomitant of trance states; in others it is an
isolated behavior. Likewise, it is variously interpreted as a possession
by god or devil, the ability to speak in a foreign tongue, or the
special gift of a supernatural tongue.

SOCIOCULTURAL ASPECTS OF GLOSSOLALIA

The social function and concomitantly the psychological significance of glossolalia appear to vary with the particular social movement of which glossolalia is a part. Several examples can be given.

R. A. Knox recounts the occurrence of glossolalia in the eighteenth and nineteenth centuries in traditional Christian groups

in which the experiential component of religious experience had been replaced by a chiefly intellectual religious practice. In this circumstance, the glossolalia was a means to reestablish an experiential base for religious faith. Concomitantly, this was during the age of the enlightenment, when rationalistic criticism of Christian faith was in vogue. Thus, the glossolalia was a "proof" of the existence of God and a validation of the believer's faith.

In the cargo cults of Melanesia, the glossolalia likewise verifies the charismatic leader's claim to authority. This seems to be a major social function of glossolalia as practiced by many shamans and priests, as reported in ethnographies.

In the staid mainline churches of America, the function of glossolalia seems to fit more into a means of protest. It can also be seen as a recurrent infusion of experiential religion into denominations that have become mainly intellectual enterprises.

By far the major practice of glossolalia and all enthusiastic behavior has been by the Pentecostal and Holiness groups. These groups are characterized by their marginal socioeconomic position in society. Here, the ecstatic behavior is both an outlet for repressed conflicts and a means of justifying one's unique position in society as a possessor of truth and righteousness.

The last variant is the function of glossolalia in middle-class Pentecostal groups who do not occupy a marginal social position. In this situation, Gerlach and Hine [10] suggest that glossolalia functions as a "rite de passage"—a technique of recruitment, a method of organization, and a means of demonstrating the claims of the movement to change people's lives. Here, the function of glossolalia is not to serve personal needs nor to serve as a mediating mechanism in relation to the larger society, but rather to serve as a mechanism for nurturance of the social movement itself.

PERSONALITY AND PSYCHOPATHOLOGY OF THE GLOSSOLALIST

A major issue concerns the personality of the glossolalist. Is glossolalia a symptom of psychopathology? Are certain personality traits associated with glossolalia? Research evidence suggests that the contradictory claims and reports are an artifact of confusion between population samples and sociocultural variables, which we have documented elsewhere [3, 17].

Knox has pointed out that eighteenth- and nineteenth-century occurrences of glossolalia were hailed by adherents as a sign of spiritual and emotional strength and health, while religious and nonreligious skeptics alike interpreted the phenomenon as a sign of emotional instability or a manifestation of emotional illness.

In the early part of the twentieth century, several psychological and psychiatric studies of glossolalists were reported. Psychological studies by Cutten, Lombard, and Mosiman concluded that glossolalists were probably emotionally unstable and that glossolalia was a regressive pathological experience.

Several clinical psychiatric studies were also published. Maeder reported a case of glossolalia in a paranoid schizophrenic, Schjelderup reported a case of tongue speaking in a neurotic during psychoanalysis, and Jean Bobon reported three cases occurring during the course of psychosis. These reports linked glossolalia to psychopathologic conflicts.

Other early reports concerned glossolalia in the context of more normal life situations, including a case reported by Oskar Pfister, one by Theodore Flournoy, and a discussion by William James. Carl Jung made allusion to glossolalia as an example of the invasion into consciousness of contents from the deepest levels of the collective unconscious as a positive preparation for integration of personality.

In our contemporary era, the clinical reports have been based on larger and more diverse samples. William Sargant and Jerome Frank allude to glossolalia as a form of regressive abreactive behavior. Weston La Barre reported an extensive case history of southern snake handlers who also practiced glossolalia. He concluded that these were examples of externalization of characterological conflict.

A series of more systematic reports have tended to support the view that glossolalia is a reflection of personality instability. Wood administered Rorschach protocols to a group of southern Pentecostals and concluded that they had unstable personality structures. Lapsley and Simpson, on the basis of interviews, concluded that glossolalia was a dissociative reaction occurring in persons with truncated personality development. Finch reported a case of glossolalia in a psychotic reaction. Klaus Thomas, in Berlin, found that all the glossolalists he saw in his suicide-prevention clinic were either preschizophrenic or had experienced psychotic episodes.

In South Africa, Vivier extensively examined glossolalists and a comparable group of controls. He found more histories of developmental conflict and life disturbances among glossolalists. Yet he concluded that in terms of personality, the glossolalists were not significantly different from the control group. Comparable conclusions were reached by Kildahl and Qualben in a study in Brooklyn.

Closer attention to sample biases was made by Paul Morentz, a psychiatrist in Berkeley. He noted that glossolalia tends to assume a different meaning in Pentecostal churches, where it is part of the expected religious ritual, in comparison to its appearance among staid mainline churches, where it is usually considered deviant behavior. Based on his interviews of 60 of the latter glossolalists, Morentz found six dominant personality patterns: (1) hostility to authority, (2) the wish to compensate for feelings of inadequacy, (3) the wish to rationalize feelings of isolation, (4) the wish to dominate, (5) strong feelings of dependency and suggestibility, and (6) wish for certainty.

Yet the two most careful and sophisticated studies yet conducted have failed to support the prior emphasis on psychopathology. Stanley Plog in Los Angeles, on the basis of an extensive battery of tests, has not found any typical personality patterns nor has he found a higher than expected rate of psychopathology. Gerlach and his associates in Minnesota, on the basis of several population samples, find no evidence of unusual psychopathology among Pentecostal adherents [10]. They conclude:

Most Pentecostals appear to be normally successful members of their families and communities . . . family relationships are more harmonious than normal in our society when all family members have had the full Pentecostal experience . . . most Pentecostals, though they are different in some behaviors are not "sick" . . . they function effectively and cope adequately. However, this does vary somewhat from group to group, and we are investigating the possibility that some groups or churches do attract more "troubled" individuals than others. It is possible that some groups in more depressed areas attract more deprived persons, or more aged lonely persons . . . it is possible that some churches stimulate in some personality types behavior which is maladaptive.

Sherrill has noted that many glossolalists in the neo-Pentecostal movements are well-adjusted individuals who are looking for an expansion of their life activities, while Sadler criticized the psychiatric inferences of psychopathology in the Episcopalian Commission report on glossolalia by noting: " . . . it is not necessarily dealing with the neurotic mind, but perhaps also with the creative, the positive aspect of the unconscious, the source of our artistic creativity."

To the reports cited above, we add our own rather unsystematic but extensive observations over a 20-year period. In brief, our observations lead us to conclude that rather than being contradictory, the various types of reports and evidence cited above indicate that glossolalia is a psychological phenomenon that bears no necessarily linear relationship with personality variables.

In common with the descriptions of Frank, Sargant, La Barre, Schwarz, and Knox, we have observed glossolalia occurring as only one of many expressions of "ecstatic," "enthusiastic," and similar "regressive" behavior, including snake handling, dancing fits, hysterical convulsions, faith healings, etc. We have typically observed these as group phenomena in lower- and lower middle-class persons in both urban and rural areas. In many of these cases, we would classify the behavior as frankly dissociative or hysterical episodes of a clinically neurotic nature. In clinical terms, we found that most of these people demonstrated overt psychopathology of a sociopathic, hysterical, or hypochondriacal nature. On the other hand, we have extensively interviewed middle-class and upper-class glossolalists who demonstrated no psychopathology. They were well-integrated, highly functional individuals who were clinically "normal." Our observations should not be construed as meaning that psychopathology is necessarily associated with social class. Rather, these class differences may reflect the personalities attracted to churches of that social strata—the same suggestion made by Gerlach and his associates and consonant with Morentz' observations. Indeed, we have found severe psychopathology among upper-class glossolalists and very normal lower-class glossolalists. We have also seen at least three cases of glossolalia in overt schizophrenic psychoses.

In taking all these observations into account, it would seem that glossolalia can be produced experimentally, as a by-product of psychotic disorganization, as a mechanism of expression of neurotic conflict, or as a normal expectation and behavior of a normal population. Thus, the phenomenon of glossolalia per se cannot be interpreted necessarily as either deviant or pathological, for its meaning is determined and must be interpreted in terms of the sociocultural context.

When glossolalia is practiced as part of the expected ritual, we would not expect to find psychopathology, whereas in situations where glossolalia is not a cultural expectation, or the group is already part of a deviant subculture, we would expect to find a correlation between glossolalia and psychopathology.

One final aspect of this problem merits comment. Many adherents of the glossolalia movement assert that the experience has made a change in their lives, has improved their style and quality of personality and life. Clinicians have been hesitant to accept such testimonials. Yet careful studies of nonpathological mystical experiences, such as in the work of Deikman, Ludwig, Underhill, and Salzman, have illustrated that mystical experience, often in a religious context, can be an integrative emotional experience that results in an altered life style with subsequent improvement in life adaptation.

In this vein, Gerlach and Hine [10] and their anthropology team comment:

There are many indications that the religious experience involved in Pentecostalism increases the willingness to take risks, and to accept technological innovations. The conversion experience is a di-

viding line between Before and After. The experience of breaking
with old religious patterns has been identified by many informants
with a willingness to break with kinship, social, and economic patterns as well. To the degree that Pentecostalism increases self confidence, inspires people to work and save, to cooperate, to take risks
and accept innovation and to break with old patterns, then it is
indeed a religious motivation for sociocultural change and economic development.

PSYCHOLINGUISTIC ASPECTS OF GLOSSOLALIA

To investigate the psychological aspects of glossolalia more
closely, we have conducted studies on a small group of volunteers,
whose speech was recorded both in normal conversation and during
glossolalia. We studied the glossolalic speech using a variety of psycholinguistic techniques. Here we shall only be able to list our
major conclusions, which are discussed at length elsewhere [3, 17].
Interviews focused on the subjects' use of glossolalia, their personality structure, and the intrapsychic uses of glossolalia. Our
conclusions were as follows:

1. Glossolalia is a learned phenomenon and can be reproduced
   by naive experimental subjects, either by imitation or upon
   request to "make up a strange language."
2. Linguistic analyses among English-speakers reveal that glossolalia is composed of basic English phonemes but employs
   a restricted linguistic code. Glossolalia is organized at a phonemic and pseudomorphemic level but lacks sememic or
   semantic structure, which differentiates it from true language.
3. Using associative techniques, glossolalia can be shown to have
   emotional meaning to subjects, although not necessarily cognitive meaning per se.
4. Glossolalia can be divided into two types: playful and serious.
   They differ demonstrably on various psycholinguistic measures and on speech spectrographic analyses. The two types
   reflect different intrapsychic functions.
5. Glossolalia represents a borderline phenomenon in the tran-

sition from inner private thought-speech to external objective language. A. similar phenomenon is typically found in the vocalizations of small children during the phase of developing cognitive mastery over the thought-speech processes. Glossolalia may thus represent a regression to an early developmental form of thought-speech function.

6. Often in glossolalia the "feeling tone" part of inner speech is transposed onto the automatic, externalized phonemic sequences, thereby allowing an individual to express feeling and emotion without revealing their manifest content.

INTRAPSYCHIC ASPECTS OF GLOSSOLALIA

Glossolalia is but one of many motor, perceptual, and cognitive functions that may occur in "peculiar" states, i.e., behavior that seems to be out of character or outside the everyday expectations of society. In both psychiatry and anthropology these states have been summed up in omnibus fashion under the terms "trance" or "possession state." Bourguignon and Pettay [2] note that in attempting to explain these phenomena in psychological terms: "A variety of hypotheses have been advanced . . . hysteria, hypnosis, nonpathological dissociation, cultural learning, social learning, histrionics, and epilepsy . . . yet these explanatory categories are themselves, on the whole, poorly understood and the argument tends to center on the question whether these states are to be considered pathological."

In his recent review, "Altered States of Consciousness," Arnold Ludwig [13] has called attention to these phenomena as "relatively uncharted realms of mental activity, the nature and function of which have been neither systematically explored nor adequately conceptualized." He defines altered states of consciousness as "any mental state, induced by various physiological, psychological, or pharmacological maneuvers or agents, which can be recognized subjectively by the individual himself (or by an objective observer of the individual) as representing a sufficient deviation in subjective experience or psychological functioning from certain general norms for that individual during alert, waking consciousness. This sufficient deviation may be represented by a greater preoccupation than usual with internal sensations or mental processes, changes in the formal characteristics of thought, and impairment of reality testing to various degrees." Ludwig goes on to note that altered states of consciousness may be produced by "a wide variety of agents or maneuvers which interfere with the normal flow of sensory or proprioceptive stimuli, *the normal outflow of motor impulses,* the normal 'emotional tone,' or the normal flow and organization of cognitive processes."

In concluding his analysis of altered states of consciousness, of which glossolalia is one instance [14], Ludwig concludes [13] that they are "final common pathways for many different forms of human expression and experience, both adaptive and maladaptive. In some instances, the psychological regression found in ASC's will prove to be atavistic and harmful to the individual or society, while in other instances the regression will be 'in the service of the ego' and enable man to transcend the bounds of logic and formality or express repressed needs and desires in a socially sanctioned and constructive way." In glossolalia we have an interesting combination of preoccupation with the thought-speech process, which interferes with both the normal flow of cognitive process (thought) and the normal outflow of motor impulses (speech).

Further theoretical elaboration has been provided by the work of Arthur Deikman [5, 6] on states of experimental meditation. Deikman focuses on the process of "*de-automatization* of the psychological structures that organize, limit, select, and interpret perceptual stimuli." The concept is derived from the work of Hartmann and of Gill and Brenman on the automatization of motor behavior. Deikman [6] concludes:

. . . de-automatization may be conceptualized as the undoing of automatization, presumably by reinvesting actions and percepts with attention. Under special conditions of dysfunction, such as in acute psychosis or in LSD states, or special goal conditions such as exist in religious mystics, the pragmatic systems of automatic selection are set aside or break down, in favor of alternate modes of consciousness whose stimuli processing may be less efficient from a biological point of view but whose very inefficiency may permit the experience of aspects of the real world formerly excluded or ignored. The extent to which a shift takes place is a function of the motivation of the individual, his particular neuro-physiological state, and the environmental conditions encouraging or discouraging such a change . . . the content of the mystic experience reflects not only its unusual mode of consciousness but also the particular stimuli being processed through that mode. The mystic experience can be beatific, satanic, revelatory, or psychotic, depending on the stimuli predominant in each case. Such an explanation says nothing conclusive about the source of the "transcendent" stimuli. God or the unconscious share equal possibilities here and one's interpretation will reflect one's presuppositions and beliefs . . . the available scientific evidence tends to support the view the mystic experience is one of internal perception, an experience that can be ecstatic, profound, or therapeutic for purely internal reasons.

From the above descriptions of the processes of deautomatization that accompany various altered states of consciousness, we can conclude, based on our own observations and the reports we have reviewed, that the uses of glossolalia are numerous. In the subjects we studied, it is used voluntarily in many secular situations to reduce tension and anxiety through a number of thought and motor pathways. The playful category of glossolalia is particularly used for the indiscriminate motor discharge of affect, as has been postulated by Rapaport [18]; that is, the individual feels a general state of uneasiness or tension or restlessness and, not knowing the cause, seeks to relieve the tension through the motor act of rapid and fluid vocalization. Glossolalia may be used in this way either consciously or unconsciously. One of our subjects claimed that during examination time he frequently would burst into tongues and usually was not fully aware of it at first. A similar phenomenon occurs when other motor acts that are used routinely to release such tension (such as tapping one's fingers or crossing legs) become so automatic and habitual that the individual is often not fully aware that he is performing them.

The "serious" category of glossolalia may also serve to aid in the reduction of tension. Some release of tension or discharge of affect can take place in the conscious awareness of a thought. In this category of glossolalia, there is a discharge of affect through thought as well as through the motor act of speaking. In addition, the encoding of the feeling tone of inner speech onto the external automatic vocalizations allows for projection of affect and tension, thereby reducing tension further. Thus, the automatic glossolalic utterances are used primarily in the serious type of glossolalia as a vehicle for the release of feelings experienced in inner speech through the audio-integument or intonational features imposed on the externalized utterances. The serious category of glossolalia provides a way of externally discharging extremely personal emotions and desires without revealing their content to others.

Subjects we interviewed often used glossolalia to entertain themselves or to relieve their boredom while engaged in rote motor tasks such as driving a car or typing. In these and other instances, subjects used glossolalia to avoid anxiety situations by blocking out the environment through listening to their own utterances and thereby altering the state of consciousness. During these times, the individual is preoccupied with listening to his vocal utterances, his breath rate becomes regular and rhythmical, and he appears relaxed to the point that his glossolalic speech becomes slurred. An altered state of consciousness probably occurs during these times. De-automatization can occur at any level in the transition from thought to speech. Thus, focusing on one's own breath sounds could alter the state of consciousness. Or the focusing of attention exclusively on the glossolalic utterance, i.e., the shape, tone, and color of the words themselves, may also alter consciousness.

In the above instances, there seems to be a degree of regression in several aspects of ego function. Indeed, in possession states or gross types of "hysterical behavior," glossolalia may occur with a marked degree of regression in most ego functions. In some glossolalists the regressive state is pathological, although in most instances of which we are speaking the regression is not pathological, but rather a regression in the service of the ego.

In the cases of students whom we studied, we were struck by the lack of regression of ego functions that occurred. These students were able to launch willfully into glossolalia with little change of consciousness or associated ego functions. Here we observe what might be termed a *highly "focal regression" in the service of the ego.*

In fact, most of the instances of glossolalia observed in the middle-class persons we have studied occur with remarkably little regression of associated ego function. The glossolalic knows his "tongue" well, that is, it is a familiar object to him. Because of this and his perception that it brings him closer to God, his "tongue" gives him security when he needs it. The restricted linguistic code of glossolalia, the predominance of vowel sounds, the egocentric "playful" quality of the utterance all suggest that glossolalia may be a focal thought-speech regression that is highly restricted to specific ego functions. Thus, glossolalia may serve to "recharge the batteries," so that the individual may continue to function or reaffirm his commitment to a style of living and adaptation to reality conflict.

In summary, our study of glossolalia reveals the vagaries of both theological and psychological interpretations that occur. The presuppositions of both theologians and scientists may skew and distort the conclusions reached. Thus, our study provides a case illustration of the value of carefully marshalling evidence and utilizing the methods of multiple scientific disciplines when faced with the evaluation of culturally atypical behavior.

REFERENCES

1. Bourguignon, E. The Self, the Behavioral Environment, and the Theory of Spirit Possession. In M. E. Spiro (Ed.), *Context and Meaning in Cultural Anthropology.* New York: Free Press, 1965.
2. Bourguignon, E., and Pettay, L. Spirit Possession, Trance and Cross-Cultural Research. Unpublished paper, Ohio State University, 1966.
3. Casey, R. L., and Pattison, E. M. Glossolalia: A Psycho-Social Speech Phenomena. To be published.
4. Currie, S. D. Speaking in tongues, early evidence outside the

New Testament bearing on "Glossis Lalein." *Interpretation* 19:274, 1965.
5. Deikman, A. J. Implications of experimentally induced contemplative meditation. *J. Nerv. Ment. Dis.* 142:101, 1966.
6. Deikman, A. J. De-automatization and the mystic experience. *Psychiatry* 29:324, 1966.
7. Devereaux, G. Normal and Abnormal: The Key Problem in Psychiatric Anthropology. In *Some Uses of Anthropology.* Washington, D.C.: Anthropology Society of Wash., 1956.
8. Eliade, M. *Shamanism: Archaic Techniques of Ecstasy.* New York: Pantheon, 1964.
9. Festinger, L., Riecken, H. W., and Schachter, S. *When Prophecy Fails.* Minneapolis: University of Minnesota Press, 1956.
10. Gerlach, L. P., and Hine, V. H. The Charismatic Revival: Processes of Recruitment, Conversion and Behavioral Change in a Modern Religious Movement. Unpublished paper, University of Minnesota, 1966.
11. Knox, R. A. *Enthusiasm: A Chapter in the History of Religion.* London: Oxford Press, 1950.
12. La Barre, W. *They Shall Take Up Serpents: Psychology of the Southern Snake-Handling Cult.* Minneapolis: University of Minnesota Press, 1962.
13. Ludwig, A. M. Altered states of consciousness. *Arch. Gen. Psychiat.* (Chicago) 15:225, 1966.
14. Ludwig, A. M. The trance. *Compr. Psychiat.* 8:7, 1967.
15. May, L. C. A survey of glossolalia and related phenomena in non-Christian religions. *Amer. Anthro.* 58:75, 1956.
16. Mischel, W., and Mischel, F. Psychological aspects of spirit possession. *Amer. Anthro.* 60:249, 1958.
17. Pattison, E. M. Behavioral science research on the nature of glossolalia. *J. Amer. Sci. Affil.* 20:73, 1968.
18. Rapaport, D. Toward a Theory of Thinking. In *Organization and Pathology of Thought.* New York: Columbia University Press, 1959.
19. Schwarz, B. Ordeal by serpents, fire and strychnine. *Psychiat. Quart.* 34:405, 1960.

Psychedelic Drugs and Mystical Experience*

WALTER N. PAHNKE

INTRODUCTION

In recent years there has been more and more publicity (much of which unfortunately has been sensationalized) about the abuse of psychedelic drugs and much less about their potential use. Throughout the complexities of this widening discussion there has been the persistent claim that these drugs could under certain conditions trigger or facilitate experiences that have been called peak, cosmic, transcendental, or mystical. Aside from being an interesting problem for theoretical research, some scientific evidence has indicated that such experiences might have therapeutic significance for psychiatric treatment. These last two points will serve as the focus for this brief survey of psychedelic drugs and mystical experience.

A BRIEF REVIEW OF PSYCHEDELIC DRUGS
AND THEIR EFFECTS

As a background for this discussion, some general information about psychedelic drugs and their effects should be reviewed. Psy-

* Based on the presentation, "The Mystical and/or Religious Element in the Psychedelic Experience," made to the Third Annual Conference of the R. M. Bucke Memorial Society for the Study of Religious Experience: "Do Psychedelic Drugs Have Religious Implications?" October 13–15, 1967.

chedelic, or "mind-opening," the term first proposed by psychiatrist Humphrey Osmond in 1957 [9], refers to a very special class of drugs that have specific and highly unusual effects on mental functioning. It is important to note that these psychological effects are quite different from those associated with tranquilizers, antipsychotics, sedatives (including alcohol), energizers, or narcotics.

As we have described in greater detail with examples elsewhere [11] [12], five major types of psychological experiences can occur when psychedelic drugs are administered to human beings.

First is the *psychotic psychedelic experience,* characterized by an intense negative experience of fear to the point of panic, paranoid delusions of suspicion or grandeur, toxic confusion, impairment of abstract reasoning, remorse, depression, isolation, and/or somatic discomfort; all of these can be of very powerful magnitude.

Second is the *psychodynamic psychedelic experience,* characterized by a dramatic emergence into consciousness of material that has previously been unconscious or preconscious. Abreaction and catharsis are elements of what subjectively is experienced as an actual reliving of incidents from the past or a symbolic portrayal of important conflicts.

Third is the *cognitive psychedelic experience,* characterized by astonishingly lucid thought. Problems can be seen from a novel perspective, and the interrelationships of many levels or dimensions can be seen all at once. The creative experience may have something in common with this kind of psychedelic experience, but such a possibility must await the results of future investigation.

Fourth is the *aesthetic psychedelic experience,* characterized by a change and intensification of all sensory modalities. Fascinating changes in sensations and perception occur: synesthesia, in which sounds can be "seen"; objects such as flowers or stones that appear to pulsate and become "alive"; ordinary things that seem imbued with great beauty; music that takes on an incredible emotional power; and visions of beautiful colors, intricate geometric patterns, architectural forms, landscapes, and almost anything imaginable.

The fifth and last type of psychedelic experience, the focus of our attention in this paper, has been called by various names:

psychedelic peak, cosmic, transcendental, or *mystical.* The psychological phenomena that characterize this experience can be divided into nine somewhat interrelated categories, as follows:

1. *Unity* is a sense of cosmic oneness achieved through positive ego transcendence. Although the usual sense of identity, or ego, fades away, consciousness and memory are not lost; instead, the person becomes very much aware of being part of a dimension much vaster and greater than himself. In addition to the route of the "inner world," where external sense impressions are left behind, unity can also be experienced through the external world, so that a person reports that he feels a part of everything that is (for example, objects, other people, or the universe), or more simply, that "all is one."

2. *Transcendence of time and space* means that the subject feels beyond past, present, and future, and beyond ordinary three-dimensional space in a realm of eternity or infinity.

3. *Deeply felt positive mood* contains the elements of joy, blessedness, peace, and love to an overwhelming degree of intensity, often accompanied by tears.

4. *Sense of sacredness* is a nonrational, intuitive, hushed, palpitant response of awe and wonder in the presence of inspiring realities. The main elements are awe, humility, and reverence, but the terms of traditional theology or religion need not necessarily be used in the description.

5. *The noetic quality,* as named by William James [2], is a feeling of insight or illumination that is felt on an intuitive, nonrational level and has a tremendous force of certainty and reality. This knowledge is not an increase in facts, but rather is a gain in psychological or philosophical insight.

6. *Paradoxicality* refers to the logical contradictions that become apparent if descriptions are strictly analyzed. A person may realize that he is experiencing, for example, an "identity of opposites," yet it seems to make sense at the time, and even afterwards.

7. *Alleged ineffability* means that the experience is felt to be beyond words, nonverbal, and impossible to describe; yet most

persons who insist on the ineffability do in fact make elaborate attempts to communicate the experience.

8. *Transiency* means that the psychedelic peak does not last in its full intensity, but passes into an afterglow and remains as a memory.

9. *Persisting positive changes in attitude and behavior* are toward self, others, life, and the experience itself.

This variety of possible effects with the same drug indicates that the mechanism is more complex than any easily reproducible drug effect alone. Most persistent researchers with psychedelic drugs have generally agreed that the exact type of experience is strongly dependent upon the necessary drug dosage, but only as a trigger or facilitating agent, and upon the crucial extra-drug variables of set and setting. Psychological set refers to factors within the subject, such as personality, life history, expectation, preparation, mood prior to the session, and, perhaps most important of all, the ability to trust, to let go, and to be open to whatever comes. The setting refers to factors outside the individual, such as the physical environment in which the drug is taken, the psychological and emotional atmosphere to which the subject is exposed, how he is treated by those around him, and what the experimenter expects the drug reaction will be.

THE EVIDENCE THAT PSYCHEDELIC MYSTICAL EXPERIENCE CAN BE FACILITATED BY PSYCHEDELIC DRUGS

What is the evidence that psychedelic mystical experiences do, in fact, occur at all? Some of the strongest indication comes from the investigators who have not encouraged or been particularly interested in such experiences, but whose patients have reported phenomena that would correspond to the characteristics listed above [6]. On the other hand, Masters and Huston [8], who are very much interested in all kinds of psychedelic experiences—including the mystical—found that only 3% (6 out of 206) of their subjects attained a complete mystical experience as measured by *their* specific definition. The most recent report from LSD researchers at the Spring Grove State Hospital in Baltimore has shown that 27% of their alcoholic patients were judged to have had the *most complete and intense* psychedelic peak experience [5].

Lack of agreement among different investigators as to the exact definition of a mystical experience is part of the reason for the difference in rates of occurrence. Any such figures need to be interpreted carefully unless a method for quantifying the experience is established, based on a standard description of the basic psychological phenomena.

Partly in response to this need, the Pahnke Mystical Experience Questionnaire [13] was constructed, based on a universal definition of spontaneous mystical experiences as recorded from all religions, ages, and cultures. The prior analysis of Stace [14] was found to be of the most help in this endeavor. An attempt was made to use psychological characteristics as free as possible from the intellectual interpretation that is inevitably conditioned by environmental factors. Each item is scored on a 0 to 5 scale of intensity. For any person completing the questionnaire, the percentage of the maximum possible score for each category can be determined. Varying degrees of completeness are possible, but to be counted as a mystical experience it was decided that the total score *and* the score in each separate category had to be at least 60%. The individual items for each category are as follows:

I. Unity
  A. Internal
    1. Loss of your own identity
    2. Freedom from the limitations of the self—feeling a unity or bond with what was felt to be all-encompassing and greater-than-self
    3. Pure awareness, being beyond the self-consciousness of sense impressions, yet not unconscious
    4. Cessation of normal impressions followed by an experience of unity in relation to an "inner world" within

       5. Fusion of the self into a larger, undifferentiated whole
       6. Unity with ultimate reality
  B. External
       7. Sense of oneness or unity with external objects and/or persons
       8. Increased intensity of particular sense impressions, resulting in experience of unity in relation to these impressions
       9. Experience of the insight that "all is one"
    10. Loss of feelings of difference between yourself and external objects or persons
    11. Intuitive experience of the essences of external objects and/or persons
    12. Felt awareness of the life or living presence in all things
II. Transcendence of
  A. Time
    13. Loss of usual sense of time
    14. Feeling that you experienced eternity or infinity
    15. Sense of being "outside of" time, beyond past and future in an "eternal now"
    16. Feeling that you have been "outside of" history in a realm where time is nonexistent
    17. Timelessness
  B. Space
    18. Loss of usual sense of space
    19. Loss of usual awareness of where you were
    20. Spacelessness
III. Positive Mood
    21. Overflowing energy
    22. Tenderness
    23. Peace or blessedness
    24. Ecstasy
    25. Exaltation
    26. Universal or infinite love
    27. Joy

IV. Sense of Sacredness
  28. Sense of wonder
  29. Sense of your own finitude in contrast to the infinite
  30. Sense of profound humility before the majesty of what was felt to be sacred or holy
  31. Sense of being at a spiritual height
  32. Sense of reverence
  33. Feeling that you experienced something profoundly sacred and holy
  34. Sense of awe or awesomeness
V. Noetic Quality
  35. Feeling that the consciousness experienced during part of the session was as real as your normal awareness of everyday reality
  36. Gain of insightful knowledge experienced at an intuitive level
  37. Certainty of encounter with ultimate reality (in the sense of being able to "know" and "see" what is really *real*) at the time of the experience
  38. You are convinced now in retrospect that you encountered ultimate reality in your experience (i.e., that you "knew" and "saw" what was really *real*)
VI. Paradoxicality
  39. Experience of paradox
  40. Sense that an attempt to describe the experience in logical statements becomes involved in contradictory language
VII. Alleged Ineffability
  41. Sense that the experience cannot be adequately described in words
  42. Feelings that you could not do justice to your experience by a verbal description
  43. You would have difficulty in trying to communicate your own experience to others who have not had similar experiences

VIII. Transiency
44. Return to your usual state of consciousness after the experience
45. Feeling that you are no longer experiencing the state of consciousness you experienced during the session

It will be noted that these items correspond to the first eight categories in the definition of psychedelic mystical experience described above. The ninth category, persisting positive changes in attitude and behavior, obviously must be measured by a follow-up questionnaire at a time interval after the actual experience. In two sets of double-blind, controlled experiments with normal volunteers, it was demonstrated that spontaneous and drug-facilitated mystical experiences are phenomenologically the same.

The first was conducted on Good Friday in 1962 [10]. Twenty theological students from relatively similar religious and socio-economic backgrounds, after medical and psychiatric screening, were carefully prepared several days before the experiment in groups of four, with two leaders for each group. All thirty participants listened over loudspeakers to a meditative Good Friday worship service in a private basement chapel, while the actual service was in progress in the church above. The experiment was so designed that half of the subjects received 30 mg. of psilocybin, and the rest, who became the control group, got as an active placebo 200 mg. of nicotinic acid, which causes no psychic effects, only warmth and tingling of the skin. From our preparation, all the subjects knew that psilocybin caused autonomic changes. Those who got nicotinic acid thought that they had received psilocybin, and suggestion was thus maximized for the control group. The drugs were administered double-blind, so that neither the experimenter nor the participants knew the specific contents of any capsule. Data were collected by tape recording, written account, the Pahnke Mystical Experience Questionnaire, and personal interview, in that order. When all the data were analyzed, the scores of psilocybin subjects were higher to a statistically significant degree in all categories than those of the control subjects.

The second series of experiments was performed at the Massachusetts Mental Health Center during 1965 and 1966 [13]. Forty carefully screened normal volunteers were selected. Most of the subjects were over 30 and held responsible professional positions in the community. The sensational publicity about LSD in the popular press added difficulties to our recruitment. We rejected more than 50% of our volunteers on the basis of medical and psychiatric history, physical examination, psychological testing, and psychiatric interview. After three hours of preparation in the days prior to the experiment, drugs were administered to four subjects at a time in a carefully prepared room with flowers, pictures of nature scenes, candle-light, and a place for each subject to recline and relax. Silence was maintained during a six-hour program of classical music. The setting was supportive, and there were no interruptions for testing during the session. We encouraged the subjects to relax and to let the music carry them. In double-blind fashion, two of each group of four subjects received 30 to 40 mg. of psilocybin, and the other two subjects, the control group, received either a threshold dose of psilocybin or an amphetamine-barbiturate combination containing 20 mg. of dextroamphetamine and 120 mg. of Sodium Amytal. The procedure seemed safe for our carefully screened normals. No one suffered apparent physical or psychological harm after a one-year follow up. In fact, all but one of the subjects said they would be willing to take the drug again under controlled conditions, perhaps sometime in the future, but not too many were eager to do so right away. Perhaps reflecting the profundity and power of their experiences, they expressed a desire for time to integrate what had been learned.

Without going into the complexities of the analysis here, it can be stated that in both experiments, the high-dose psilocybin group had a statistically higher number of mystical experiences than did any of the control groups. Using the 60% level of completeness on the questionnaire as the definition of a mystical experience, only one control subject out of a combined N of 30 controls for both experiments had a mystical experience, whereas at least 35% of the high-dose psilocybin subjects (total $N = 30$) did so in each of the research projects.

IMPLICATIONS FOR PSYCHIATRY

Human experiments have been performed with synthesized mescaline during the last 50 years, but it was not until the introduction of LSD in the 1940's that interest in psychedelic drugs as an experimental psychiatric tool became widespread. These drugs, especially LSD, have been used for a variety of purposes in psychiatry: production of "model psychosis"; research on brain enzymes; change in sensory modalities, cognitive processes, and psychomotor coordination; and study of the range of human emotion. However, it is the potential for therapeutic usefulness that is most germane to our present discussion.

In attempts to harness the psychedelic experience for psychotherapeutic effectiveness, three major methods have evolved: psycholytic therapy, psychedelic chemotherapy, and psychedelic peak therapy [1]. In psycholytic therapy, the aim is usually the uncovering of unconscious material that can be psychodynamically analyzed both concurrently and in subsequent therapeutic sessions. This type of therapy is relatively long-term, with multiple sessions over time and usually with a small dose of the drug. In psychedelic chemotherapy, the major emphasis is on the psychedelic drug session itself, during which intensive psychotherapy may or may not be carried out. There is minimal preparation and follow-up therapy. A single session with a relatively high dose of the drug is the usual practice. Sometimes hypnosis is combined with this method (so-called hypnodelic therapy). The major differences between psychedelic chemotherapy and psycholytic therapy are number of drug sessions, amount of therapy outside the drug sessions, and drug dosage. In psychedelic peak therapy, one major aim is the achievement of a peak or mystical experience; also essential are concentrated psychotherapeutic preparation for the psychedelic drug session and intensive follow-up therapy to help with the work of integration. Preparation involves not only the usual psychotherapeutic concerns but also the religious ideas and feelings of the patient. The latter are especially important during the work of follow-up integration, when there is a persistent demand on the part of the patient to interpret the experience in a way that is intellectually satisfying. The patient's own religious framework is usually a useful aid in this effort.

At the American Psychiatric Association meetings in May, 1968, three research teams reported their results using a combination of LSD and psychotherapy in the treatment of alcoholics. Ludwig et al. [7] and Johnson [3], who used varieties of psychedelic chemotherapy with varying degrees of actual psychotherapy, reported negative results. Kurland et al. [5], who used psychedelic peak therapy, reported positive results so far in a study not yet completed at the Spring Grove State Hospital. The most striking finding of Kurland's group was that those patients who have the most intense and profound mystical experiences are the ones who do best in terms of follow-up evaluation for as long as 18 months after therapy. Psychedelic peak therapy is at present being investigated by the same group for potential therapeutic usefulness in ongoing research projects at the Maryland Psychiatric Research Center with alcoholic, narcotic addict, neurotic, and terminal cancer patients [4]. Results thus far have been quite promising. It is important in evaluating such conflicting reports to note that the method of procedure is quite different with psychedelic chemotherapy and psychedelic peak therapy.

IMPLICATIONS FOR RELIGION

Mystical experiences can be interpreted in religious language, but not necessarily. Whether or not a mystical experience is a religious experience depends upon one's definition of religion. The definition of religion could be made so specific and narrow that most mystical experiences by the above definition would not be included. Conversely, all religious experiences are not necessarily mystical. The conviction by some individual experiencers that psychedelic mystical experiences are religious has led to the formation of four formal psychedelic churches who use some sort of psychedelic drug as their sacrament: the League for Spiritual Discovery (LSD), founded by Dr. Timothy Leary; the Neo-American Church, founded by psychologist Arthur Kleps; the Native American Church, established more than 50 years ago by the American Indians; and the Church of the Awakening, founded by two physicians, Drs. John and Louisa Aiken. These organizations no doubt will face many legal challenges in the future.

Organized orthodox religion has reacted in general to the phenomenon of psychedelic mystical experience with suspicion. Yet with increasing numbers of serious people becoming interested in psychedelic drugs as a possible means for spiritual growth, the Church might do well to find ways to help persons integrate their psychedelic mystical experiences in a healthful way. The framework and symbology of religion seem naturally suited as an aid to the understanding of these experiences. Religious themes and symbols many times are an important part of the content of psychedelic experiences. One of the most important applications of psychedelic drugs may be as a valuable tool for research in the psychology of religion for a more scientific understanding of the dynamics and psycho-physiological mechanisms of the mystical experience. In addition, an excellent opportunity is provided for a controlled study of the effects of such experiences over time on stable, well-adjusted, adequately functioning members of society who might volunteer for such psychedelic drug experiments.

IMPLICATIONS FOR SOCIETY

A major cause for social concern about psychedelic drugs has been the growing black market and inevitable psychiatric casualties from their increasing uncontrolled use, although it must be admitted that we still have no reliable figures on the incidence or rate of occurrence of harmful effects. However, the dangers of abuse must not be allowed to cloud the solid scientific evidence that when psychedelic drugs are administered under controlled medical conditions (as has been the case in several large-scale research projects in recent years), permanent adverse effects have been quite rare. At the Spring Grove State Hospital, for example, more than 300 patients have been treated with LSD without a single case of long-term psychological or physical harm directly attributable to the treatment, although there have been two transient post-LSD disturbances that have subsequently responded well to conventional treatment.

Yet the growing social problem of the black market in psychedelic drugs remains. The most reasonable and effective method of attacking this problem is through education and research. People need to know the facts, free from sensationalism. Increased research is urgently needed to understand more about what these drugs can do and how they work.

CONCLUSIONS

We now have the technology for studying and facilitating experimental mystical experience, but much more must be learned about this fascinating phenomenon. The only way the psychedelic mystical experience will ever find a constructive and socially acceptable use in an inter-disciplinary way in both religion and psychiatry is through an expansion of research. Such research must be sensitive to the religious dimension as a powerful factor in human life. Whether or not we can harness this potential for the mutual benefit of religion and psychiatry remains, at present, an open question.

REFERENCES

1. Abramson, H. A. (Ed.). *The Use of LSD in Psychotherapy and Alcoholism.* Indianapolis: Bobbs-Merrill, 1967.
2. James, W. *The Varieties of Religious Experience* (Modern Library Edition). New York: Longmans, Green, 1902, pp. 371–72.

3. Johnson, F. G. LSD in the Treatment of Alcoholism. Paper presented to the American Psychiatric Association meeting in Boston, Massachusetts, May 15, 1968.

4. Kurland, A., Pahnke, W., Unger, S., and Savage, C. Psychedelic therapy (utilizing LSD) with terminal cancer patients. *J. Psychopharm.* 1968.

5. Kurland, A., Unger, S., Savage, C., Olsson, J., and Pahnke, W. N. Psychedelic Therapy Utilizing LSD in the Treatment of the Alcoholic Patient: A Progress Report. Paper presented to the American Psychiatric Association meeting in Boston, Massachusetts, May 15, 1968.

6. Leuner, H. *Die Experimtelle Psychose.* Berlin: Springer Verlag, 1962.

7. Ludwig, A., Levine, J., and Stark, L. A Clinical Evaluation of LSD Treatment in Alcoholism. Paper presented to the American Psychiatric Association meeting in Boston, Massachusetts, May 15, 1968.

8. Masters, R. E. L., and Huston, J. *The Varieties of Psychedelic Experience.* New York: Holt, Rinehart & Winston, 1966, p. 307.

9. Osmond, H. A review of the clinical effects of psychotomimetic agents. *Ann. N.Y. Acad. Sci.* 66:418, 1957. Also in *LSD: The Consciousness Expanding Drug.* D. Solomen (Ed.). New York: Putnam, 1964, pp. 128–51.

10. Pahnke, W. N. *Drugs and Mysticism: An Analysis of the Relationship between Psychedelic Drugs and the Mystical Consciousness.* Harvard University Ph.D. thesis, 1963. Results are summarized in Pahnke, W. N. The contribution of the psychology of religion to the therapeutic use of the psychedelic substances. In *The Use of LSD in Psychotherapy and Alcoholism.* H. A. Abramson (Ed.), *op. cit.,* pp. 629–52.

11. Pahnke, W. N., and Richards, W. A. Implications of LSD and experimental mysticism. *J. Relig. Hlth.* 5:175, 1966.

12. Pahnke, W. N. LSD and religious experience. In *LSD, Man, and Society.* R. C. DeBold and R. C. Leaf (Eds.). Middletown, Conn.: Wesleyan U. Press, 1967, pp. 60–84.

13. Pahnke, W. N., Salzman, C., and Katz, R. Experimental data in preparation.

14. Stace, W. T. *Mysticism and Philosophy.* New York: Lippincott, 1960.

The Scrupulosity Syndrome

GEORGE MORA

HISTORICAL BACKGROUND

On March 6, 1691, at Whitehall before the Queen, Bishop John Moore of Norwich preached a sermon on "religious melancholy" in which he made reference to persons plagued by guilt feelings or "dread of those Punishments which he hath threatened to inflict on unrelenting sinners" despite "their . . . sincere love of God"; these same people experience "a flatness in their minds . . . which makes them fear, that what they do, is so defective and unfit to be presented unto God, that he will not accept it"; they are overwhelmed by "naughty, and sometimes Blasphemous Thoughts" which "start in their Minds, while they are exercised in the Worship of God" despite "all their endeavours to stifle and suppress them." Unfortunately, these thoughts are anything but easy to overcome, as "the more they struggle with them, the more they encrease"; furthermore, "they are mostly good People . . . for bad men . . . rarely know any thing of these kind of Thoughts." For the treatment of such a condition he suggested "gentle Application of such comfortable things as restore the strength, and recruit the languishing Spirits that must quash and disperse these disorderly tumults," and finally he advised "not to quit your Imployment . . . For no business at all is as bad as too much; and there is always more Melancholy to be found in a Cloyster, than in the Market-place" [13].

163

As far as is known, this is perhaps the first publication specifically dedicated to the subject of scrupulosity [2, 10, 15, 16, 25]. Of course, this is not to imply that prior to then sincerely devoted people were not afflicted with obsessive thoughts, especially of impure and blasphemous nature as well as of unworthiness. But the fact that there was no exclusive focus on it until the end of the seventeenth century is an indication that the problem had not acquired special importance until that time.

From the modern viewpoint, influenced by the dynamic view of the personality, it is understandable that the problem of scrupulosity may have become noticeable in the context of the personal religion of the Protestant ethic. The Puritan outlook toward life had necessarily resulted in the disturbing awareness of much (thoughts and actions) that did not fit the high standards of cleanliness in exterior habits and in inner life. In the Middle Ages, the community had provided a healthy outlet for feelings of guilt, through the extensive use of public atonement to God, as outlined in the numerous handbooks of penance, called Penitentials [1, 18]. In a culture as theocentric as the medieval one, it is likely that a number of emotional disorders were included in the list of "sins" dealt with by the Penitentials, thus offering ample provision for the open expression of guilt feelings related to them [26]. This practice can be traced back to the rite of exomologesis of the early Christians, which involved self-humiliation of the penitent, dressed in sackcloth and given to austere diet, in order to win the compassion of the congregation and gain personal salvation. Previous to that, it is enough to remember that the history of the Hebrew people is all centered on the vicissitudes of the relationship between God and his chosen people, highlighted by the dynamics of sin, divine wrath, and repentance. Even the personal religion of the Greeks and Romans, which, together with that of the Jews, contributed to the foundations of the Christian world, provided an outlet for the public expression of emotions related to sin (especially *hybris*, that is, arrogance of thoughts toward the divinity) through the impressive rituals of the Asklepeians [6, 19].

In modern times, the Reformation and the Counter-Reformation, by emphasizing the individuality of conscience and of worship, had the effect of depriving men of a cathartic means of expression of guilt feelings, while at the same time slowly building up the elaborated architecture of sins and repentance of the casuistry. In the nineteenth century, following the revolution of criticism in philosophy and of social institutions in politics, the Hegelian and the Marxian approach tended to corrode the very basis of the Judeo-Christian tradition. The churches of various denominations, as well as orthodox Jews, were patently unprepared to deal with these utterly revolutionary trends, which, as far as the study of the mind is concerned, resulted first in materialism and then in the advent of dynamic psychiatry at the beginning of our century.

Today, after several decades of mutual distrust and misunderstanding, the validity—and differences—of some basic points relevant to psychology and religion are generally accepted: the superego stemming from individual and societal unconscious in contrast to moral conscience based on conscious will; human actions as resulting from moral freedom in the boundaries of the biologically determined individual [23]; revealed religion as part of the reality of the patient, to be duly acknowledged and constructively used for therapeutic purposes. Official statements on the part of the psychiatric professions do not hesitate to emphasize the positive value of religion [8, 9], while, on the other side, clergymen of all faiths are increasingly engrossed with the relevance—on theoretical and practical grounds—of dynamic psychology for their pastoral functions.

CURRENT KNOWLEDGE OF THE SYNDROME

For all this mutual effort at an integrated view of the personality, inclusive of its moral and religious aspects, relatively little gain has been made in the field of scrupulosity. Perhaps this statement should be made less pessimistic by clarifying that a considerable gap has occurred between (1) the knowledge of the personality of the scrupulous person and (2) the type of intervention—sacramental, therapeutic, or both—most effective in the handling of these people.

The Personality of the Scrupulous Person

It is a fact that scrupulous persons can be found in all kinds of religions, though they are most often found among the Roman Catholics, especially among those inclined to interpret Catholicism from the Puritan perspective. The reason for this is rather complex, perhaps mainly due to the unconscious feelings of rebelliousness and antagonism that the very rigid structure of the Catholic Church —unnecessarily and unwisely made more frightening through the mirage of Hell—arouses in many. The very ritual of repentance, confession, and absolution, which in itself should lead to a joyful rebirth in Christ in the sacrament of penance, may instead enhance the feeling of guilt in a personality predisposed to a masochistic orientation. While this applies as well for all the other Christian denominations, in Judaism a similar feeling of guilt can stem from the fear of breaking God's law, as expressed in centuries-old customs and rituals.

It is indeed universally recognized by psychiatrists, and accepted by clergymen [5, 11, 27], that the scrupulous person, rather than having a "delicate" conscience, tends to be mistrustful of himself and of others—including the many confessors he has "tried"—and to cling to one conviction, that of his own sinfulness. At the basis of his obsessive thoughts—as we have learned from psychoanalysis— are deep, unconscious, infantile wishes of sexuality and aggression which cannot be accepted by the ego and which therefore are distortedly expressed through the symptom of scrupulosity. Typically, these people, in their perfectionistic urge, are never sure of having gone through the entire list of their sins in the confessional, and they consider themselves unworthy of receiving the comforting benefit of the divine Grace. As they consider themselves martyrs vis-à-vis the endless demands of their conscience, one would expect that they should accept whatever the priest—who represents God—

decides on the matter of their sins and proper penance. Instead, they do not hesitate to argue with the priest that their confession has not been completed and that therefore they are not ready to receive Communion. Aside from verbal expression of dissatisfaction with the priest's decision, they express even greater criticism by returning over and over again to the confessional in the vain attempt finally to find solace for their obsessive minds. Thus, clinically they present the characteristic picture of the passive-aggressive, sadomasochistic personality, which is included in the chapter of the disturbances of the total personality [3, 7, 14].

The best analogy to this kind of behavior is that of the child continuously returning to the mother because he is not satisfied with what he receives from her. This opens the way to the consideration of the early development of scrupulous people. Invariably, one finds that their rigid outlook toward life in thoughts and in actions—of which their religiosity is a typical expression—has its roots in early disturbances of their personality. Quite often, as a child, the scrupulous individual was raised in a family in which his parents presented definite problems, from schizoid behavior, depression, and delinquent acting-out to severe marital (especially sexual) problems, while all along giving the impression in the community of a "normal" family with typical (including religious) middle-class values. It is no wonder that, being raised in an environment basically deprived of love, such a child is adversely affected by the negative image presented by his parents, while, at the same time, he is expected to present a good image of himself in the community. The sexual feelings of the normal oedipal period are distorted, the aggressive feelings toward the parents are turned toward himself, and in the course of time his guilt acquires pathological proportions. The only way for the individual to cope with this situation is to isolate as much as possible his overwhelming anxiety related to the guilt through obsessive thoughts of unworthiness and compulsive rituals of purification.

These symptoms, as one would expect, become more prominent at adolescence, when biologically and culturally the sexual and aggressive urges gain impetus. As this coincides with the crisis of

identity that eventually results in the choice of a vocation, it is no
wonder that—in certain cases, at least—the selection of the religious
vocation may be influenced by the religiosity stemming from a
scrupulous personality. It is a fact that scrupulosity is a rather frequent symptom, quite often the first one, in seminarians suffering
from emotional disorders. The reason for it is that such a symptom
is "acceptable" by the seminarian's conscience in the religious context of the community life. In my experience, in every case where
it persists for some time despite the usual counseling offered by the
spiritual director, it can be traced to earlier years. Thus, the seminary life in itself does not cause the disturbance; rather, it simply
brings it to the surface and provides "justification"—through the
emphasis on purity of life—for a preexisting symptom. Quite often
this symptom is simply one of a constellation that includes masturbation, poor personal relationships, and other symptoms and finds
its real cause in loneliness and insecurity, as recent studies have
indicated [12].

Whether it affects a layman or a future clergyman, the essence
of the symptom of scrupulosity remains the same, except, of course,
for the compound danger of a pathological influence of the future
pastor's emotional disturbance on his parishioners: basic frustration toward excessive demands of the conscience and toward the
sterile repetition of the same pattern of guilt, expiation, and ac-
cumulation of more guilt; projection of aggressive impulses onto
God, who is viewed from the narrow perspective of guardian of
morality; neurotic use of religion, which, degraded to empty rituals
and formulas, covers up the real meaning of the symptom. This
real meaning is constituted by the over-concern with one's own
"spiritual" life at the expense of involvement with others, either
in the basic dual modalities of the "I-thou" (such as between husband and wife, parent and child, teacher and pupil) or in the
multiple modalities of community and social life.

The scrupulous person gives the impression of spending his life
in preparation for the time when he will finally be at peace with
God; but in the meantime—and this can take the best part of his
life—he refuses to engage himself in life; that is, he escapes the

existential meaning of his life. Surely, in considering the early onset of his emotional disorders in childhood and adolescence, much of the guilt that the scrupulous person experiences stems from repression of unconscious sexual and aggressive wishes; that is, it is independent from consciously sinful actions. Even if a school of psychology, reasserting what some German psychiatrists (notably Heinroth) claimed during the Romantic period [17, 28], states that all guilt is real inasmuch as it stems from the repression of the superego (rather than of the id) and, consequently, that all neurotics are real sinners in need of religious penance [21, 22], the main consensus of those active in the field of religion and psychiatry is for a combined effect of conscious and unconscious guilt [24]. In such a way, consideration is given to the psychiatric treatment of scrupulous individuals, while at the same time maintaining the validity of the sacrament of penance, based on an act of will of the penitent in the context of the doctrine of free will, as traditionally held by churches of any denomination.

Intervention—Sacramental and Therapeutic

Having thus far sketched the personality of the scrupulous person in general, it is necessary, of course, to know more concerning the individual person in order to provide the proper type of intervention. Even in the absence of statistical data, it is safe to say that most of the cases of scrupulosity fall into the obsessive-compulsive type of personality. In cases of rather acute onset, perhaps due to particular external circumstances, in a personality not giving evidence of long-term established pathology, a supportive type of counseling by the pastor himself may be sufficient to achieve improvement. As invariably the pastor is the first to identify the scrupulous individual, in the confessional, it is his duty to have at his disposal some quick notions of how to categorize his penitent. In any case, he will have to acquire an idea of the type of personality he is dealing with, in terms of actual functioning of the penitent at home and in society, presence of other psychiatric symptoms, way of relating to others, previous occurrence of the same symptom, and, if possible, at least a glimpse of his early development, especially in terms of the crisis of adolescence. As all this cannot be accomplished in the limited time and atmosphere of the confessional, it is advisable that a pastor who repeatedly hears the confession of an alleged scrupulous penitent attempt to see him at length in the sacristy or in his office—even more than once—so that he can gain some insight concerning the severity of the penitent's pathology and, of course, after a few sessions, have the opportunity to learn how he (or she) relates to him.

Some years ago, I tried to define the characteristics of the transference situation that may develop between the pastor and the penitent in the context of such counseling [20]: a psychotherapeutic action consisting of a mixture of cathartic relief "from below," that is, expression of emotions related to basic conflicts, and an ontological reinforcement "from above," that is, a clarification of the all-embracing love of God for men and of the sanctifying role of Grace in the brotherly spirit of the Church—quite opposite to the penitent's view of a tyrannical God and of an alienated world. As indicated in my earlier paper, the type of relationship established between the penitent and the pastor is very much influenced by the type of relationship that the penitent experienced in the past toward parental and, later, authority figures; quite often it was a highly ambivalent mixture of love and hate. Conversely, the pastor will have to check constantly his own feelings, in order to avoid developing a condemning attitude toward the penitent. This danger can be minimized not only by awareness acquired through previous experience of the pastor in working with other scrupulous patients, but also by a knowledge of basic human psychology and pastoral counseling that he may have learned in his studies, in postgraduate courses, and in field work, which nowadays are becoming increasingly available in churches of all denominations.

This does not mean to say that the pastor should turn into a psychotherapist, but simply that he should be aware of certain basic psychological phenomena, even at the preliminary stage of assessment of the personality of his penitent who presents signs of scrupulous behavior. Fortunately, in many cases of mild scrupulosity, a few sessions of this informal counseling are all that is needed. Whether, in similar circumstances, the priest should not be hesitant in imposing penances, as has been suggested, remains questionable [20]. Coming back to what was said initially, it is true that in the Middle Ages, and even in antiquity, the community provided outlets for public expression of guilt and penance; but guilt was then mainly public, in the context of a shame-ridden society and of a theocentric vision of man and his world, which is quite different from the guilt-ridden modern society and from the man-centered view of the modern world, in which guilt has become the private affair of the individual conscience.

Unfortunately, in other cases of severe scrupulosity, the situation is far from being so simple. The counseling offered by the pastor either is not accepted or is unable to modify the situation to any extent; the penitent cannot relate and continues to present the same behavior; quite often, it is clear that his adjustment to life has been very marginal, as the penitent lives alone, isolated, only able to follow a self-imposed strict routine that impinges on any spontaneous expression of love and charity. The question that should arise spontaneously, even in the mind of a layman such as the pastor, is, of course, what would happen to this person if this strict routine could be removed from him. The answer is clear: the person would not be able to function, since, in psychological terms, this routine represents for him the best defense. As a matter of fact, people presenting this sort of personality would clinically be diagnosed as schizoid, if not simple (or ambulatory) schizophrenic.

On the surface, the case of the pastor who has identified severe psychological symptoms in his penitent could be considered rather simply as a referral to a professional person. In reality, things do not go so smoothly. First of all, the penitent, especially if severely disturbed, may resist any thought of requiring professional help by insisting that he is only motivated by a religious urge to salvation. Second, the penitent may abandon the pastor who has advanced the idea of professional help to "try" another confessor, in the hope that this other one may accept the solely religious interpretation of the trouble. Third, even if the penitent accepts referral to a professional person, the question arises of who this person should be. Most often, he would be a psychiatrist, a psychologist, or a person from another field—including a clergyman—who is known for his experience and interest in dealing with scrupulous patients. That the therapist be of the same religion as the patient is not, in my opinion, strictly necessary, though belonging to the same religious denomination may decrease the patient's resistance to therapy.

The important points for the therapist are the following: (1) he should have established some sort of working relationship with clergymen in the community, so as to facilitate the process of referral of the patient, of on-going communication, and of discharge of the patient back to the referring pastor; (2) he should quickly assess the personality of the patient, even with the help of psychological tests, in order to formulate a therapeutic program; (3) this therapeutic program quite often should consist of individual treatment based on a combination of expressive and repressive therapy; and (4) in any case, the therapist should maintain a positive view of the penitent's religion as an intrinsic part of his reality, quite often important for its supportive role when void of neurotic distortions. Aside from the selective and temporary use of psychopharmacological agents on the part of medical therapists, other forms of treatment should be considered, such as consultation with clergymen, especially those extensively involved in pastoral counseling, as spiritual directors in seminaries. It has also been suggested that group therapy, after a series of individual sessions, could be beneficial.

SUMMARY

In contrast to the exclusive emphasis on long-term individual therapy in the past, today's psychotherapeutic means offer more variety and flexibility in line with the different needs of the patient and the manifold collateral forms of assistance provided by the community. A great deal of this, however, is still in the early stages of development and is largely a matter for the future. It is for this reason that the initiatives taken by various groups toward common work of clergymen and professionals in the field of mental health —through meetings, workshops, special publications, and so forth— should be supported and enhanced by all those genuinely interested in the integration of modern psychological principles with the concept of man as traditionally held by religion. On a more practical and modest basis, all this may eventually result in the alleviation of much suffering on the part of the scrupulous individual, who may finally understand the basic theological truth that no one can be tempted beyond his limits, thus opening the way to a sincere acceptance of his own personal destiny and of the salutary effect of Grace as provided by the sacrament of confession and penance.

REFERENCES

1. Anderson, G. C. Medieval Medicine for Sin. *J. Relig. Hlth.* 2:156, 1963.
2. Barbaste, A. Le scrupule et les données actuelles de la psychiatrie. *Rev. Ascet. Myst.* 28:3, 1952.
3. Bowers, M. K. *Conflicts of the Clergy.* New York: T. Nelson, 1963.
4. Corcoran, C. J. D. The management of scrupulosity. *Insight* 2:17, 1964.
5. Demal, W. *Pastoral Psychology in Practice.* New York: P. J. Kenedy, 1955.
6. Dodds, E. R. *The Greeks and the Irrational.* Berkeley: University of California Press, 1951.
7. Fenichel, O. *The Psychoanalytic Theory of Neurosis.* New York: W. W. Norton, 1945.
8. Psychiatry and religion: Some steps toward mutual understanding and usefulness. *Group Advance. Psychiat.* [*Rep.*] 48, 1960.
9. The psychic function of religion in mental illness and health. *Group Advance. Psychiat.* [*Rep.*] 67, 1968.
10. Grutton, H. Essai de psychologie pastorale sur le scrupule. *Suppl. Vie Spir.* 48:95, 1959.

11. Hagmaier, R. G., and Gleason, R. *Counseling the Catholic.* New York: Sheed & Ward, 1959.
12. Herr, V. V. Mental health training in Catholic seminaries. *J. Relig. Hlth.* 5:27, 1966.
13. Hunter, R., and Macalpine, I. *Three Hundred Years of Psychiatry.* London: Oxford University Press, 1963.
14. Laughlin, H. P. *The Neuroses.* Washington, D.C.: Butterworth, 1967.
15. Lauras, A. Scrupuleux et obsédés: étude psychiatrique. Cahiers Laennec 20:3, 1960.
16. Mailloux, N. The problem of scrupulosity in pastoral work. In *Proceedings of the Institute for the Clergy on Problems in Pastoral Psychology.* New York: Fordham University Press, 1956.
17. Marx, O. A re-evaluation of the mentalists in early 19th century German psychiatry. *Amer. J. Psychiat.* 121:752, 1965.
18. McNeil, J. T., and Gamer, H. M. *Medieval Handbook of Penance.* New York: Columbia University Press, 1938.
19. Meier, C. A. *Ancient Incubation and Modern Psychotherapy.* Evanston, Ill.: Northwestern University Press, 1968.
20. Mora, G. The psychotherapeutic treatment of scrupulous patients. *Cross Currents* 7:29, 1957.
21. Mowrer, O. H. *The Crisis in Psychiatry and Religion.* Princeton, N.J.: Van Nostrand, 1961.
22. Mowrer, O. H. *The New Group Therapy.* Princeton, N.J.: Van Nostrand, 1964.
23. Plé, A. Moral acts and the pseudo morality of the unconscious. *Cross Currents* 9:31, 1959.
24. Pope Pius XII. *On Psychotherapy and Religion.* Washington, D.C.: National Catholic Welfare Press, 1953.
25. Snoeck, A. La pastorale du scrupule. *Nouv. Rev. Theol.* 79:371, 1957.
26. Telfer, N. *The Forgiveness of Sins.* Philadelphia: Muhlenberg, 1960.
27. VanderVeldt, J. H., and Odenwald, R. P. *Psychiatry and Catholicism.* New York: McGraw-Hill, 1952.
28. Zilboorg, G. *A History of Medical Psychology.* New York: W. W. Norton, 1941.

Religious Conversion

LEON SALZMAN

INTRODUCTION

Conversion experiences have accompanied mass movements of all kinds—religious, social, and political. Due to the charismatic quality of the leader or the magnificence or value of the message, some people experience a dramatic conviction of belief in the individual or in his beliefs. Phenomena of this kind were widespread prior to the Christian era and abounded in primitive societies. The test of the value of the conversion was not one of validity but of consistency with the prevailing ethic. Prior to a science of psychology capable of dealing with such phenomena, these experiences were examined entirely within the framework of the prevailing philosophy and religious systems. They were judged entirely on theological grounds and were considered to be products of either God or the devil.

Psychological theory has introduced an additional consideration, which is the recognition of the dynamic elements in a conversion experience that may be an attempt to resolve personal problems through the medium of religious symbolism. Such conversions may be related to religious feelings but may not represent a true religious experience. Phenomena such as mysticism, fanaticism, and asceticism can be explored in this way as well.

As the theologian has become psychologically more sophisticated, there is a greater reluctance to automatically accept every claim of a spiritual experience as valid. This has not diminished the growth of real religious feelings; rather, it has intensified the conviction about valid religious attitudes. In an atmosphere of increasing intellectual sophistication and profound knowledge of the universe and its operating principle, primitive, fundamentalist views of religious experience can only be maintained in an atmosphere of total ignorance. Psychology has a solid place in the theological armamentarium, not only in terms of mental health but also for the examination of certain theological phenomena.

The problem of belief and the development of trust can be explored from a psychological framework now that we can recognize that trust is not inborn, like an instinct, but develops out of the growing experiences of the infant in relation to his physical and human environment. Trust must be one of the earliest developments in the infant, since he is so utterly dependent on the benevolence of his environment for survival. He has no capacity to recognize that when mother is visually or audibly absent she will return in due course. Only a repeated set of experiences of such a predictable order ultimately develops sufficient trust that this will occur. When the predictability is absent, we can recognize the most far-reaching effects in the order of fear, mistrust, insecurity, anxiety, suspicion, and so forth. It is clear that trust does not grow out of single or multiple experiences, but out of a large number of experiences extending throughout the life of a person. Yet its beginnings are laid down in early infancy, and these can prejudice and influence one's later attitudes and beliefs. It is from such beginnings that trust, faith, and, ultimately, religious feelings grow.

Fanatical belief, however, or pseudo trust, can develop from the need to establish some security in an insecure world and to overcome grave doubts and morbid fears about oneself and others. Under these circumstances, a person adheres to a belief out of desperation rather than from conviction, and out of fear rather than from positive feelings. The difference can be seen in mass movements in which devotion or dedication are attempts to establish some security or belonging through a sharing of hates and negative attitudes toward the world, in contrast to those mass movements that are inspired by high ethical principles and loving attitudes toward the world. Converts, dedicated disciples, and fanatics can exist in both groups. The conversion process, as will be noted, is greatly dependent upon what one is converted to and toward what goals and purposes [7, 11].

In evaluating true religiosity versus spurious religiosity, it is important to recognize many aspects of the activity of the individual in addition to his professed spiritual beliefs. Phenomena that were considered to be of divine origin in earlier years are now recognized as being derived from discoverable physical causes. This is becoming increasingly true of phenomena derived from psychological sources. Consequently, the social scientist may have a great deal to offer the theologian in elucidating the dynamics and motivations of human behavior in spiritual areas.

DEFINITION OF CONVERSION

In its broad sense, conversion has long been a subject of psychological interest. The motivation and mechanics of change—and conversion is primarily this—have always interested philosophers and psychologists. Religious conversion, however, has remained in the realm of philosophical speculation and clerical mystification except for the investigations of certain brave and enlightened clerics, such as Sante de Sanctis [4], and a few psychologists such as William James and others [1, 3, 8–10, 12, 13]. Most clerical writers see the phenomenon as a "visitation," or a profound mystical experience incapable of scientific investigation. Consequently, their studies have made few contributions to psychology, although the detailed descriptions by converts of their own experiences have frequently supplied vital psychological data [2].

Religious conversion is a specific instance of the general principle of change in the process of human adaptation. Conversion is a generic term for change and generally implies a drastic alteration of a former state. In the physical sciences, the term *conversion* is used to indicate an extreme change, such as converting water into steam by heat. Freud used the term to convey the alteration and translation of psychic energy into somatic channels producing physical symptoms. This characterizes some hysterical phenomena. Conversion simply means a change; however, in theological terms it has been used in a special sense to imply a marked alteration of one's spiritual state through a superior power, generally meaning a Godhead. It is a development that implies some spiritual or mystical significance. However, we know that some conversion experiences in a theological framework can be due to forces other than the spiritual.

In the course of human development, many changes occur. Some are mild and gradual, while others are sudden and dramatic. Many individuals, because of severe thwarts, traumas, or defects in maturation, develop problems that require drastic solutions and major readjustments. We may therefore find in the lives of these people experiences that are dramatic, explosive, and far-reaching, and that are attempts to solve pressing personal and interpersonal difficulties. They may have no spiritual significance, yet they can be expressed in religious language or symbolism.

Most change—possibly all—is gradual in its development; but since it culminates in a specific moment of alteration, it may seem to the observer to be an instantaneous, unexplained, and mysterious event. Conversion cannot be regarded as a sudden or dramatic event, although under extremely hazardous and life-endangering circumstances profound changes may occur with only limited background and preparation.

Much confusion exists concerning the phenomenon of religious conversion. Each writer describes it according to his own inclination and prejudice. There is no definition that is applicable to the variety of phenomena that the word *conversion* is used to describe. For the purposes of this paper, I shall consider conversion to be any change of religion or of moral, political, ethical, or aesthetic view that occurs in the life of a person either with or without a mystical experience, and that is motivated by strong pressures within the person. As I am considering it, the experience is not identical with "religious experience," though the two may surely coexist. Though religious experience may be defined in a number of ways, it often seems to involve cosmic feelings, states of rapture, and mystical phenomena, and it can be likened to the "ecstatic absorption" that occurs when a dissociated tendency reaches awareness and threatens the integration of the personality. This may or may not be followed by schizophrenic process. It should be noted that insight often occurs with such profound feelings of expansion and cosmic identification and is often considered to be a religious experience. This phenomenon is extremely interesting and needs to be studied further to illuminate the problems both of insight and of change. In this paper, the conversion experience will be examined from a purely psychological point of view, regardless of whether the change produced a new religious belief or a greater involvement in the old affiliation. Studying the conversion process means considering where the convert went, that is, what he converted to; the factors that caused him to change; and why he went where he did. It is also necessary to examine his behavior after the conversion in order to understand more fully what effect the conversion has had on his beliefs and attitudes and in order to determine the value and significance of the experience, since verbalizations are often very deceiving. "By their acts, so shall ye know them," is a profound Christian aphorism, rich in implications about conscious and unconscious behavior. In understanding the conversion process, we must be able to distinguish between particular pieces of behavior and total character structure.

TYPES OF CONVERSION

Using this definition of conversion, we must first consider the conversions that are conscious, deliberate, and calculated. We may call these expedient conversions; they represent attempts to deal with realistic problems in such a way as to obtain material advantage or to sustain oneself in the face of certain disaster. While this conveys a good deal of insight into the person's character structure, it is not the result of an inner struggle nor of deep philosophical or moral inquiry. It is a practical solution that may occur in all spheres of living—moral, ethical, intellectual, political, and spiritual. For purposes of definition and clarity, I suggest two major types of conversion.

Progressive or Maturational Conversion

This type frequently occurs in the course of real maturing; it takes place when a person, after a reasoned, thoughtful search, adopts new values and goals that he has decided are higher than those he abandoned. It occurs in reasonably normal people, and when it is a religious conversion, it represents the achievement of the ultimate in the humanistic religions—positive fulfillment of one's powers, with self-awareness, concern for others, and oneness with the world. It occurs as the result of an achievement of cosmic identification as an outgrowth of maturity in the humanistic religions. It is also a possible result of reaching maturity after psychoanalytic therapy. It may be a political or ethical conversion, or it may be a spiritual conversion quite outside the framework of religion. I call such conversions progressive in the sense that the movement is forward in terms of personality development, and permits greater maturity. The struggle involved usually concerns the dynamics of "love" as opposed to "care," and it represents the person's endeavor to expand and to express his creative, positive, kindly attitudes toward his fellowman and the world at large. This conversion can be called a conjunctive one, brought about by a lessening of anxiety; it is an integrating, maturing development in the life of the person. The conversion of George Fox illustrates this type. It is equivalent to the experience in therapy when one finally notices something that produces massive changes in the personality structure. In psychotherapy it is called insight—but it is analogous to the conversions of religious people who achieve higher integration based on their conception of God. It is also like the experience of satori, which is arrived at in Eastern religions.

Regressive or Psychopathological Conversion

This type of conversion is the main subject of this paper. I approach this question as a psychiatrist and scientist who considers the phenomenon as arising from natural causes and therefore comprehensible on natural grounds. Obviously, not all events or phenomena can be adequately explained by present-day scientific skills. When they cannot, one may be tempted to call upon supernatural causes and personify them in deistic terms. As long as we can acknowledge that such labels signify that no cause has been established, we can feel free to use them.

Theologians have stated, regarding the conversion process, that "man's extremity is God's opportunity." This appears to be particularly applicable to the regressive conversion, for it is a highly charged, profound, emotional experience that occurs during attempts to solve pressing and serious problems in living, or to deal with extreme, disintegrating conflicts. It may take the form of a mystical, emotional change in religious affiliation or a sudden, dramatic enthusiasm within the framework of the person's own group. It is a pseudo solution and is likely to occur in neurotic, prepsychotic, or psychotic people, although it may also occur in presumably normal persons who are faced with major conflicts or insuperable difficulties. Thus, while it is often considered a psychotic development, it is not necessarily so. However, because it is brought about by increasing anxieties and has a disjunctive effect on the personality, it may either precipitate or be part of the psychotic process. At the same time, because the conversion experience may include some conjunctive elements and because of its defensive nature, it may ward off a psychosis.

I designate this type of conversion as regressive only in the sense that such conversions produce changes that are defensive solutions and that partake of the characteristics of psychopathological phenomena. While the motivations and conflicts may seem to be similar to those in the progressive conversions, the dynamics deal with affects other then love, and the outcome is manifestly different.

I do not mean to convey the impression that one kind of conversion is good and the other bad, or that one has greater merit than the other. My object is to study those conversions that, under psychological investigations, reveal in their manifest and covert forms the characteristics of a destructive, disintegrating process, as opposed to those that constitute a constructive and integrating process.

Descriptions of conversion range from those viewed as a normal process occurring in adolescence (Pratt [10], Starbuck [12], and Thouless [13]), to those seen as an emotional struggle away from sin towards righteousness (James [8], de Sanctis [4], Boisen [2]).

In 1924, Freud [6] wrote a short piece on religious conversion in response to a letter from an American doctor describing his conversion experience. The conversion followed an intense emotional experience in the morgue, when the doctor had, as an intern, seen a "sweet old lady" on a slab. In analyzing the experience, Freud noted that the conversion occurred after an intense reactivation of the early oedipal hatred of his father. The hatred succumbed to a powerful opposing current and ended in complete submission to the father in the form of Christ. Freud noted that the conversion had relevance to the writer's hatred of his father. In his short paper, Freud touched on the dynamic process involved and went to the very core of the conversion process, although he did not document it in further writings.

Earlier writers on conversion recognize that aside from the elated mystical experience, profound struggle and torment are involved in the process. However, none of them has attempted to distinguish between different kinds of conversions in terms of their motivations or the dynamics of the struggle preceding the conversion experience. The theologians have not been concerned with the impetus or motivation, provided that the proclamation of faith conformed to their concept of the religious doctrine.

In view of the increasing influence of psychological theorizing, which is based on a growing body of solid data to substantiate it, there is a continued uneasiness in dealing with all conversions outside of the Pentecostal or Fundamentalist sects, where they are encouraged and welcomed. Theologians are often too aware of the pathological elements in these experiences, and in spite of their desire to affirm such experiences, they are loath to do so publicly.

Clinical Examples

Shortage of space permits the inclusion of only a few clinical examples of regressive conversion.

Mr. B, whose problems included a suspicious, hostile attitude toward the world, particularly toward the Catholic Church, had converted to Catholicism when he was 22 years old, after years of indecision. His history included a running battle with his father, which continued until the latter's death, in which Mr. B was indirectly involved. His father was a tall, rigid, and autocratic Jew who favored Mr. B's older brother. This brother was tall like his father, and more worldly than Mr. B, who was small and weak and felt that he was despised by his father. Even though he was very successful in school, he did not feel that he had his father's respect, and Mr. B. strove, by increasingly rebellious and antagonistic activity, to force recognition from his father. While his father followed the forms of the family religion, his attitude toward it was contemptuous, and he was without any real values or ethics. Mr. B was idealistic and was troubled by his father's hypocrisy. For a while he tried conscientiously to conform to the ethics of their religion, but the atmosphere of his family and community made this impossible. His mother was a weak, impotent, and mildly accepting figure in the family, who dedicated her life to trying to make peace between the patient and his father; her place in the patient's life seemed to have been relatively unimportant.

The estrangement between the patient and his father continued to grow, and their relationship was finally completely ruptured when the son converted to Catholicism. The conversion, which he had contemplated for a long time, took place when he was rejected by a Jewish girl friend. In part, the conversion resulted from a warm friendship he had with a priest who assumed a foster-father role toward Mr. B. Several years after he joined the Church, Mr. B. married a Catholic girl.

Mr. F. had been raised as a moderate Protestant. He began therapy while contemplating converting to the Catholic Church and entering a monastery to become a member of an ascetic order. Shortly before he began therapy, he detailed his plans for conversion in a long letter to his family. The letter was full of both subtle and direct hostility, directed primarily at his father. Mr. F's family had always been quite antagonistic to the Catholic Church; thus, his plans represented a double blow, since he proposed both joining the Church they disapproved of and removing himself forever from contact with them. Before proceeding further, however, he began psychotherapy, and after some time decided against this conversion. Mr. F. is now studying for the Protestant ministry.

A young man of 22, who had been having considerable difficulty with himself and his family, left college after one day's attendance. He decided to become an artist and began to paint and to mix with the beatnik crowds. He used marihuana and narcotics and spent much of his time in what he called "desire and fear." He was antagonistic toward his family and felt that the whole world was hostile and selfish. He left his wife after getting involved in Hindu mystical teachings. Unfortunately, this patient could only be seen briefly, so the details about his early life are sketchy. However, he described his conversion experience in great detail. He was seated with two friends. One was painting while the other was reading a religious tract. Suddenly, he felt himself being emptied of all desire, after trying to cope with angry feelings he noticed were passing through his mind. At the same time, he was also being freed from fear. He felt liberated and at peace with himself. He thought God had entered into him, and while he had no words to describe the experience, he knew it was a Christian God as personified by Christ. This feeling passed quickly, and he felt that he must preselytize and decided to go West. He had a reconciliation with his wife, and after visiting his father he was taken to a mental hospital. His appearance was striking. He was outwardly calm, peaceful, and unruffled, and smiled freely and amiably. He expressed no hostility, anger, desire, or fear, even while describing a hostile, competitive world. In the course of the interview, however, though he claimed he was not angry, I suggested that his eyes, voice, and tone indicated that he was, in fact, quite angry. He denied this, though this impression was confirmed by six other observers. At one point, when he was speaking loudly and in an irritable manner, it was suggested that he was angry. He replied that while he could kill somebody, he was not angry. I indicated that to kill not in anger was even more hostile than to kill in anger. He refuted this hotly by quoting Hindu scripture.

THE DYNAMICS OF THE CONVERSION EXPERIENCE

It is clear that hatred, resentment, and hostile, destructive attitudes seem, in each of the cited cases, to have been involved in the preconversion experiences. While many observers have noted these emotions, they have not seen them as the focus of the preconversion struggle, nor have they quite seen conversion itself as an attempt to deal with them. Pratt [10], James [8], Starbuck [12], and others [3, 9, 13] see conversion as the result of an intense struggle within oneself, but none of them recognizes the forces of hatred operating in the struggle. Freud, however, suggests this in his brief paper on the subject [6].

Another indication of the dynamic involvement of this type of conversion with hate is provided by revival meetings led by "hell-fire and damnation" preachers who spout hate, not love, and inflame the congregation with threats of eternal damnation and with descriptions of the most vile and hateful consequences of sinfulness. One may well ask what is stirred up in the audience, love or hate? What leads to the sudden urgency to be converted? It seems to me that in such cases there is an activation of hateful feelings to such a frightful extent that it can be mollified or made acceptable only by the conversion experience.

The following description of such a situation was written by a minister:

I remember well back in 1936 attending a large church service in Toronto, Canada, in which an outstanding preacher spent an entire sermon on a blistering attack on the members of the theological faculty of the seminary I was attending (they were unfit, not Christians, and so on), and at the end of the sermon gave an "altar-call" (a call to those in the congregation who felt converted and wanted to become professing Christians). A number of people did respond to that "call"—were converted, presumably. Could I venture the supposition that the dynamics of that "call" were in some way tied up with the "hate" manifested by the preacher—and "appealed" to similar feelings of the ones who responded?

Such hateful feelings can be mobilized under other circumstances as well. The mass conversions that took place during the Crusades could, to a certain extent, be considered a product not only of the actual threat to life of the infidel, but also of the atmosphere of hatred, destruction, and violence that accompanied the Crusades.

The overt behavior after a conversion to some extent reveals the character of the conversion experience. I believe this is the one single factor that gives us the best clue to the meaning and character of the experience. The postconversion behavior of the constructive conversion is markedly different from that of the regressive one. In the last conversion reported in this paper, the young man abandoned his previous interest in art and set out to roam with a group of friends to "spread the word." He had no plans for working or supporting himself and in essence was laying the groundwork for going either to jail or to a hospital. He was certainly not preparing himself to carry on the humanistic mission about which he verbalized.

The postconversion behavior characteristics of regressive conversions are, perhaps, exaggerated in mystical conversions. These are as follows: (1) the convert has an exaggerated, irrational intensity of belief in the new doctrine; in many converts, however, though they may remain in the new faith, the ardor doesn't continue at the same high level, as indicated by the high percentage of backsliding cited by Starbuck [12]; (2) the convert is more concerned with the form and doctrine than with the greater principle of his new belief; (3) his attitude toward his previous belief is one of contempt, hatred, and denial, and he rejects the possibility that there might be any truth in it; (4) he is intolerant toward all deviates, with frequent acting-out by denouncing and endangering previous friends and associates; (5) he shows a crusading zeal and a need to involve others by seeking new conversions; and (6) he engages in masochistic and sadistic activities, displaying a need for martyrdom and self-punishment.

Many of these characteristics represent the antithesis of a loving, kindly solution to the problem. They indicate that the attempt to channel hatred into acceptable forms has been only a partial solution, for the hatred becomes evident in many devious ways. Thus, the convert, although zealously sought after by the group, is largely unaccepted by the members of it because of his extreme rigidity and his moral and doctrinaire excesses.

The conversion experience seems to be an attempt, usually by especially gifted, sensitive, and basically decent people, to solve a problem of great magnitude in their lives. The religious solution is tried by these who have spiritual goals and whose philosophy encompasses magic and extreme dependency on strong, omnipotent figures. The conversion can occur in a sudden, overwhelming way and produce a dramatic or revivalistic change, but usually there are long years of deliberation and preparation, with growing feelings of impotent fury and helplessness. Occasionally with adults, and often with adolescents, the inner struggle with the problem of hatred toward the father or toward father symbols—that is, authority—results in overwhelming anxiety and can result in the conversion experience, whether this experience is psychotic, neurotic, or "normal" [5].

REFERENCES

1. Ames, E. S. *The Psychology of Religious Experience.* Boston: Houghton Mifflin, 1910.
2. Boisen, A. T. *The Exploration of the Inner World.* New York: Harper, 1936.
3. Coe, G. A. *The Psychology of Religion.* Chicago: University of Chicago Press, 1916.
4. de Sanctis, S. *Religious Conversion: A Bio-Psychological Study.* London: Kegan Paul, Trench, Trubner, 1927.
5. Furgeson, E. H. (Ed.). Special Issue on Religious Conversion. *Past. Psychol.* Part I, 16:156, 1965; Part II, 17:166, 1966.
6. Freud, S. A Religious Experience (1925). In *The Complete Psychological Works of Sigmund Freud* (Std. ed.). London: Hogarth Press, 1955, Vol. V.
7. Hoffer, E. *The True Believer.* New York: Mentor Books, 1951.
8. James, W. *The Varieties of Religious Experience.* New York: Longmans, Green, 1902.
9. Leuba, J. H. *A Psychological Study of Religion.* New York: Macmillan, 1912.
10. Pratt, J. B. *The Religious Consciousness: A Psychological Study.* New York: Macmillan, 1926.
11. Salzman, L. The psychology of religious and ideological conversion. *Psychiatry* 16:177, 1953.
12. Starbuck, E. D. *The Psychology of Religion.* New York: Scribner's, 1903.
13. Thouless, R. H. *An Introduction to the Psychology of Religion.* New York: Macmillan, 1923.

PART III
CLINICAL ASPECTS OF THE
MENTAL HEALTH OF
RELIGIOUS PERSONNEL

This section focuses on those special needs and problems that require the particular attention of the clinician who treats religious personnel. Although human nature and human problems are universal in large part, religious beliefs and vocations do color patterns of illness, assessment, and treatment.

Christensen reviews the clinical studies on the mental health of clergymen, concluding that mental illness among the clergy is neither more nor less than among the general population. However, he points out that the ministry attracts certain personality types, and that the ministry poses particular stresses leading to characteristic conflicts. Esau and Cox present their clinical experience in treating ministers' wives and families. They note the paucity of clinical studies in this area and suggest some areas of particular concern for preventive mental health. McAllister summarizes a series of studies on members of religious communities. He spells out the particular emotional needs and strains of living in such communities and points out the need for mental health resources. Cox and Esau outline the specific problems involved in assessing candidates for religious service. They stress that general clinical diagnosis is not enough, for church agencies need assistance in defining both strengths and weaknesses and "goodness of fit" for particular kinds of service. Bowers concludes with a seasoned

189

resume of the typical problems encountered in the psychotherapy of religious patients. She notes the obvious difficulties,
offers practical suggestions, and recounts the rewards that can
come to both the therapist and the patient.

The Mental Health of Clergymen

CARL W. CHRISTENSEN

INTRODUCTION

We live in the midst of social unrest, overpopulation, urban renewal, war, inflation, LSD, and "the pill." We live in a time of questioning and change. Now, as in the past, clergymen are called upon to interpret the meaning of this turmoil and provide standards by which changing cultural values and social mores may be evaluated. But the Christian Church, itself, is engaged in a process of self-appraisal and reorientation regarding its meaning and function. Albeit the clergy are expected to provide dynamic leadership and counsel for people beset with problems, it is not surprising that there should be some casualties and that an occasional minister should falter or succumb to a mental disorder under the stress of his responsibility. When mental disorders occur in professional persons, it is a source of concern, since the consequences can affect people over whom they wield considerable influence.

Only a few, relatively isolated psychiatrists have been interested in the mental health of ministers. Those psychiatrists who are concerned with the mental disorders of the clergy naturally focus on the diagnosis and treatment of psychopathology. A few have been active in preventive medicine as it pertains to the mental health of ministers. Psychiatric research relating to mental disorders of clergymen is empirical in nature and is usually derived from the incidental data of clinical experience. There is general agreement concerning the effect that predisposing causes, the stresses of the religious vocation, and religious beliefs and practices have upon the types of mental disorders of ministers. Those readers interested in the literature on the subject are referred to the excellent annotated bibliographies of Menges and Dittes [4] or Meissner [3].

INCIDENCE OF MENTAL DISORDERS AMONG CLERGYMEN

Any attempt to determine the prevalence of mental disorders among religious personnel can, at best, yield only vague approximations. The few studies that have been made are limited in scope. Morgan [5], for example, polled 26 state hospitals by questionnaire, and concluded that the number of hospitalized clergymen was equivalent to other patients of the same faith. Southard [6] studied the incidence of mental disorders in several professions and decided that acute psychological reactions were no more common in the clergy than in other professions. I believe that the incidence of mental disorders found in clergymen is essentially the same as in the general population. However, I also think it significant that certain reaction types tend to predominate in those clergymen with mental disorders. I have reported some of these observations previously [2].

At this writing, I have seen 294 seminarians, graduate ministers, and missionary candidates, mostly for a diagnostic evaluation. Of the 13% considered psychotic, all but one were suffering from some form of schizophrenic reaction, mainly the paranoid type. The lone exception was diagnosed as a psychotic depressive reaction. Of the rest, 38% were considered to be psychoneurotic reactions, of which about half were suffering from depression, and the remainder were seen as having some form of character disorder. In the latter category, passive-dependent-aggressive personality trait disorder, homosexuality, and sociopathic personality trait disorders predominated. I believe that this distribution indicates, first, that the ministry attracts individuals whose basic character structure predisposes to these conditions, and, second, that once in the ministry, the particular stresses encountered lead to or precipitate maladaption.

While the evidence is far from conclusive, it is interesting to note that certain types of pathology seem more prominent in some religious denominations than in others. Alcoholism is a continuing problem with Episcopalian and Roman Catholic priests, while it is essentially nonexistent among Methodist clergymen. The latter tend to have, in my experience, a higher incidence of psychoneurotic depressive reactions and passive-dependent personality trait disturbances than do Protestant clergy of other denominations. Homosexuality, exhibitionism, and voyeurism occur throughout the ministry but seem especially high with Episcopalians and Roman Catholics. Of 35 Roman Catholic clergymen seen in the private practice of psychiatry, 9 were homosexuals, 12 were schizophrenic, 6 had passive-aggressive-dependent personality trait disturbance, 3 depressive reaction, and 1 each of manic-depressive psychosis, psychotic depressive reaction, obsessive-compulsive reaction, anxiety reaction, and compulsive personality. (I am indebted to Dr. James E. Vanderbosch for these statistics.) The more liberal clergymen tend to have a higher incidence of psychoneurotic and psychophysiological reactions, while the fundamentalist clergymen seem prone to psychoses and more severe character disorders. However, the significance of these empirical observations requires further study and elaboration.

PREDISPOSITION

It is self-evident that clergymen are subject to the same vicissitudes, in the course of their maturation, as we all are. While there are still some neuropsychiatrists who question the importance of early environmental influences upon the developing personality structure, most dynamic psychiatrists agree that environmental factors determine the characteristics of the adult personality structure. There is a difference of opinion as to the relative importance of specific factors and the degree to which they exert an influence. However, most authorities agree that the family is the single most important force molding the character structure. From the histories of the patients it is possible to make some generalizations concerning the family environment from which clergymen come. Generally, the more disturbed family backgrounds are reported from patients with the severest pathology.

Invariably, the mother is the major dominating influence in such homes. Her attitude toward her husband is usually hostile, rejecting, and domineering. Frequently, she turns to hard work and to the church to find the love and acceptance she wants but can't accept. Interestingly enough, although there is much marital disharmony, divorce is relatively rare and separation uncommon. Apparently the continuation of the marriage meets conscious and unconscious needs. The mother's attitude toward the children is, at best, ambivalent. Often she is rejecting and frustrating under the guise of concern. Case histories of clergymen suffering severe pathology reveal instances of provocative acting-out of the mother lasting into the adult life of the potential clergyman. As she is sexually frigid, her sons become forbidden sexual objects toward whom she is provocatively seductive but ultimately rejecting. In contrast, the histories of ministers suffering from psychoneurotic difficulties have mothers who were frequently described as being prudish about sexual matters.

Father was generally regarded as a nonentity. In the more severe cases, father had died at or before adolescence of the future clergyman, or had withdrawn emotionally from the family. When he did interact, it was usually with anger and rejection. Chronic alcoholism was common. Religion was seldom a resource for the father, who tended to use his work as a substitutive means of gratification. Rarely were his sons able to make a dominant identification with him, and when they did the father introject was usually a depreciated one.

In general, the families belonged to the lower or lower-middle socioeconomic classes. Among the Protestant clergy, the severest pathology was predominantly in those coming from a rural or small-town environment. Clergymen coming from larger urban centers were theologically more liberal and tended to suffer from the middle-class illnesses—psychoneurotic reactions and psychophysiological reactions. Most ministers with mental disorders use religious beliefs in an attempt to solve intrapsychic conflict. When this fails, or when the stresses are too great, anxiety develops, leading to symptom formation.

SPECIAL STRESSES OF CLERGYMEN

With the possible exception of medicine, no other profession is subject to such prolonged, intense, and often paradoxical tension as is the ministry. It is not surprising, therefore, that with a given predisposition, added stresses should precipitate psychopathology. Daniel Blain [1] has discussed these in some detail, hence it is only necessary to mention a few by way of example.

Perhaps one of the most common sources of tension is inherent in the profession itself. No other profession makes such difficult claims upon its membership as does the Church upon its clergymen. The minister is expected to go forth from his seminary and function successfully as a theologian, philosopher, businessman, politician, educator, preacher, public relations expert, and psychotherapist, with relatively little educational preparation. The congregation, also, expects him to be expert in these matters. If he fails, he may not be openly vilified, but he is often relegated to obscurity. Competition for the higher ecclesiastical positions is intense and usually undercover, since the clergyman is not expected to have ambition. The minister is supposed to go where he is told and do what is demanded without protest or argument. A rigidly hierarchal church places the clergyman in the ambiguous position of having to be a dynamic leader to his congregation and a humble supplicant to his superiors. The resulting tensions may eventually take their toll.

Financial strain is chronic with clergymen. It is presumed that the minister will not be concerned with "worldly goods." Traditionally, he is dependent upon the beneficence of the congregation. This places him in a difficult situation. Socially his status is high, while economically it is low. He may be the recipient of certain fringe benefits, but the constant receiving of charity can undermine his self-respect. The ministry is, essentially, the only profession that fails adequately to reward its membership financially for their work. Such deprivation frequently has its effect upon their families, leading to resentment and rebellion, particularly with the children. In addition, there are restrictions placed upon personal pleasures and emotional expression. Freedom and privacy are often limited. The minister and his family are required to deny normal interactions, as they often believe they must present an idealized image to their congregations. Furthermore, the clergyman is often the subject of the unconscious needs of his congregation. Religion frequently emphasizes the symbolic and therefore readily lends itself to fantasy, of which the minister is the object. Such displaced feelings may occasion a counterreaction on the part of the minister, causing untenable situations. These, and other stresses, in their cumulative effect, may produce a breakdown of ego defenses, resulting in acute reactions and symptom formation. The specific symptoms will be dependent upon the predisposing factors, current stress, and individual ego defenses.

Recently, however, there have been some further sources of stress that are worthy of consideration. Today the Christian Church is engaged in a rather agonizing reappraisal of itself in relation to society. At the same time, society is in process of changing its values and mores. As a result, there is an increasing awareness among the clergy that to provide dynamic leadership requires involvement. To those who used the ministry as a refuge, these changes are often anxiety-producing. With others, it may cause anger. Occasionally, clergymen whose unconscious use of the religious vocation was a reaction-formation against their own hostile rebellious feelings against authority become active in various aspects of social action. It is not uncommon that such behavior becomes overdetermined, resulting in acting-out.

CHARACTERISTIC PROBLEMS OF CLERGYMEN

As the evidence accumulates, I am impressed by the relative constancy with which clergymen tend to have certain specific types of pathology. The reasons why are complex but worthy of some consideration.

I think the most common single factor leading to anxiety and conflict in the clergy is the inability to love and be loved. I believe this is caused by the fact that they were unloved as infants, were loved ambivalently, or were loved conditionally. Those who were unloved tend to develop psychotic reactions or severe character disorders. They are often attracted to the religious vocation in an effort to make up this lack by receiving God's love and the love of their congregation. Unfortunately, their past experience is such that they cannot accept either. Their ministry suffers as a consequence, since they seek symbolic gratification to the detriment of their relationships with others. Those individuals who were loved ambivalently during their developmental years grow up doubting their ability to love and be loved. They are inclined to develop psychoneurotic reactions or some type of character disorder. As clergymen they seek assurance for their doubts, but since they can't accept the evidence of their relationships, they develop various symptoms. Depression and psychophysiological reactions seem to predominate within this group. Finally, those individuals who were the recipients of conditional love are liable to perceive love as a threat to their sense of identity. To be loved means giving up being themselves. They seek, in the religious vocation, the unconditional love of infancy. They never find it. The result is commonly a depressive reaction or a hostile acting-out in the form of passive-obstructionism. In each of these instances, the self-concept is depreciated and the body image is distorted. Consequently, a fantastic ideal self is conceptualized—that of being the perfect clergyman. Failing to measure up to the fantastic standard, they react with guilt, a sense of inadequacy, and anger, which finds expression in a need to atone or prove themselves. The ministry thus becomes self-centered rather than object-centered. Under such circumstances, they identify with rather than empathize with deprived people, resulting in rebellion against authority.

The current social unrest and change furnishes an opportunity for clergymen to unconsciously use the social situation for their own unconscious needs. But it has another effect. It has caused increased preoccupation with the question of identity. More and more the clergyman has to find his sense of identity not only in terms of his subjective self, but in relation to his objective self, that is, as a functioning member of society. In the past this was relatively easy to do within the framework of an essentially static church. Today this is not easy, since the demands of the culture require action on the part of the clergy. Many ministers lack the objective sense of identity that expresses the function of the subjective in terms of environmental interaction. This type of identity confusion is different from that described in borderline psychoses, in which there is confusion of the subjective sense of identity. The resulting difficulty of function often leads to frustration and, consequently, anger, which is introjected to find an outlet in depression.

In keeping with the general culture, another very common area of conflict among the clergy is sexuality. Partly because of the identity confusion, the clergyman may use sex in an attempt to verify himself as a functioning adult. But because this comes into conflict with aspects of the Christian ethic, he may experience guilt and shame and have to deny and repress his normal feelings and reactions. On the other hand, his need to prove himself can lead him to put aside old values in favor of licentiousness. With the development of "the pill" and changing social mores, there is increasing confusion concerning values of sexual behavior. While there has always been some sub rosa sexual behavior, in the past four or five years the action has increased. For example, the male seminarian is more active sexually and finds willing partners among his female counterparts on campus. The married seminarian away from his family during the week may find a sexual partner on campus. Extramarital affairs among the graduate clergy seem to be increasing.

In the past, society's attitude toward hostility favored covert expression, which encouraged repression or suppression of anger and hate with the frequent development of behavior based upon reaction-formation. The resultant intrapsychic conflict caused such symptoms as passive-obstructionism or psychophysiological reactions. With the changes taking place in both the church and society, opportunities for expression are more directly available. If the hostility against authority is an expression of unconscious rage against rejecting parents, the resulting behavior is often overdetermined. Judgment is impaired, so acts of civil disobedience are condoned that can ultimately negate the basic altruism of social concern. This social change has other consequences. In the past, the religious vocation was frequently a haven for those men with strong unfulfilled dependency needs. Within the structure of the church, these clergymen could make an adaption. Now, with the change toward a more dynamic church, these clergymen find their dependent adaption threatened. The resulting anxiety may precipitate a depressive reaction.

SUMMARY

The occurrence of mental disorders among clergymen is essentially the same as among the general population, although certain reaction types seem to be attracted to the ministry. Special stresses of the ministry added to a developmental disposition may occasion acute or chronic reactions. The changing social structure has its effect on the ministry, increasing the stress and possibly causing a change in the type of mental disorder common to the clergy.

REFERENCES

1. Blain, D. Fostering the mental health of ministers. *Past. Psychol.* 9:9, 1958.
2. Christensen, C. W. The occurrence of mental illness in the

ministry. *J. Past. Care* 13:79, 1959; 14:13, 1960; 15:153, 1961;
17:1, 1963; 17:125, 1963.
3. Meissner, W. W. *Annotated Bibliography in Religion and
Psychology.* New York: Academy of Religion and Mental
Health, 1961.
4. Menges, R. J., and Dittes, J. E. *Psychological Studies of Clergymen.* New York: T. Nelson, 1965.
5. Morgan, L. Mental illness among the clergy: A survey of state
mental hospitals in america. *Past. Psychol.* 9:29, 1958.
6. Southard, S. The mental health of ministers. *Past. Psychol.*
9:43, 1958.

The Mental Health of Ministers' Wives and Families

TRUMAN G. ESAU AND RICHARD H. COX

INTRODUCTION

Due to the paucity of material written on the subject, this chapter will be approached from the clinical point of view. It will therefore, of necessity, reflect the authors' personal clinical experience. The clinical psychological picture of the minister's wife is unique. The expectations and responsibilities are different from those of the wife of almost any other professional one could consider. It is rarely possible for the minister's wife to be the unseen and unheard spouse of the professional person. She is expected by a multitude of persons to meet their individual expectations and prejudices regarding the religiosity and service role demanded by them. One might question the motivation and developmental history by which a woman chooses to be the wife of a minister. Our observations tend to indicate that as an adolescent she has sought a status identity that arises out of the sociocultural religious framework that assumes a basic denial of emotional and physiological gratification. She must be willing to accept a life of financial, personal, family, and many other kinds of sacrifice. The attendant aura and belief in future reward for such sacrifice is assumed to be more than adequate for this self-denial. She becomes the subject of sacrifice both voluntary and involuntary. What is voluntary sacrifice to one woman will not be so to another. The degree of personal psychological need and ability for sublimation will help to dictate the degree to which her sacrifice is pathological. The sacrifice extends, however, beyond the material and monetary to the willingness to spend many evenings alone due to her husband's involvement in church activities. This results in a loneliness that cannot be compensated for even by friends, for the minister's wife is not allowed many close friends, and certainly very few among the local constituency. This is the case because the minister's wife is not allowed to "play favorites," nor can she take the risk of being on one side or the other in any theological or administrative controversy. She is essentially unable to live as an individual, and, therefore, her need gratification is reduced. It is assumed that she will find her gratification vicariously through her husband and by a rather indefinable and highly spiritualized personal religious experience. She becomes one who authenticates her husband's role as the godly man in the community [7]. It is assumed that by being a good woman she adds to his stature as a good man. The minister's wife often finds herself involved considerably beyond her depth, without the understanding of the congregation. She has been made a leader and is frequently forced into an environment beyond the capacity she has developed from her training and experience and background. It is assumed too often that, although she is not a seminary graduate, by virtue of being married to a minister, she has been trained to perform the functions of a minister's wife. She is therefore not allowed to utilize her own talents and capabilities where she feels best as a person, but is cast into a role of expectancy, whether she has the capabilities for such or not.

For many women, this role represents a way of life that is highly satisfactory, in which they find considerable sublimation. Some see it as a "first lady" position and therefore feel themselves "queen of the congregation." Some also find it most gratifying to be in the position of bringing insight to their husbands regarding the nature of their ministries and the expression of their persons. Typical items discussed regarding the pastor's wife, as observed in the literature [1, 2, 3, 4] (which it must be acknowledged is limited), point to her role as counselor, confidant, worker with other women, force in the community, hostess, teacher, and executive in church functions such as women's groups and denominational women's activities. It is apparent that much of this role has been written by tradition, and she falls into it without personal choice. For women whose narcissistic needs require prominence and a career without the full companionship of marriage, the role of minister's wife may offer some fulfillment. In traditional conservative Protestant circles, the only role of prominence that a woman is allowed is that of the minister's wife. It would be very significant if we could know how many of these same wives would have become ministers if female ordination had been acceptable in the history of the American Protestant movement. The complexity of this whole subject increases with the overlapping of gratification that can arise from the role with the deprivation of other gratifications that result from role ambivalence, i.e., wife-mother-church leader. By virtue of being such an important person in the congregation, the minister's wife may also come to feel that she lives somewhat of a fishbowl existence. The loneliness mentioned before may be a daily experience, but she's more often observed than accompanied in this plight. She is subject to much loneliness, for though she is allowed to be the confidant of many, she does not feel comfortable in allowing herself to be a person in return. On the other hand, with the gratification that arises from being in the public eye and being seen as an important person comes also the inevitable criticism if things are not done as the congregation desires. Her children, therefore, are subject to criticism on the basis of their behavior, their dress, and their performance. Not only does she face criticism of herself and her children, but she must also deal with criticism directed at her husband. She thus is made a recipient of criticism that she may not feel about him herself. This provides added stress to the marital situation, which may already be pressed by the exhaustive commitment that the couple must make to the work. These external criticisms can place the minister's wife in real jeopardy as a person if she cannot see them in the context of their meaning for the congregation. If she personalizes them, her marriage will be in trouble.

The deeper complicating factor for her is the danger of becoming hostile and resentful, for in this respect she may feel guilty for appearing to contradict what she believes God has "called" her to do [4].

It is difficult to talk about the minister's wife without also including the children, who share many of the role expectations described above. On the one hand, they are provided with a place of prominence in the eyes of many. They are subject to indulgence to the point of abuse at times by the well-meant gifts and solicitations of the congregation. Coupled with this are the rather great expectations that the pastor's children should be able to perform at an exceptional level because of their close relationship to the pastor and, in turn, to God. Furthermore, the opportunity for the members of the minister's household to benefit from a frank expression of the meaning of these stresses and requirements is often deprived them because of the religious expectation that one should accept the role with grace. The consequences of deviant behavior in the minister's child are much more grave than for the general population. Because the child's behavior in some sense is expected to authenticate the minister's adequacy as a professional person, the child early comes to recognize that deviance can threaten his father's position in the community.

In addition, the minister's family must be mobile. Transfers and changes in pastorates sometimes occur every few years, leading to considerable insecurity for both the wife and children. Multiple moves, various and often inadequate homes, financial concerns, shifts in schooling, loss of friends, and a lack of "roots" characterize this rather nomadic existence.

PATHOLOGY

Our observations at this point will turn to psychopathology, for this is the major area of our experience, having been clinicians to the minister's wife and family and thus able to observe the effects of the roles and the maladaptive mechanisms used to deal with them. In our experience, the most frequently encountered clinical syndrome in the minister's wife is that of hostile dependency. One cannot understand this hostile dependency without also perceiving something of the typical balance in the marital relationship between the minister and his wife. The counterbalancing of passive-aggressive and passive-dependent characteristics is a typical theme observed in such marriages. In many respects it can be said that many minister's wives see their role as a fulfillment of aggressive needs. The wife can find fulfillment and identification in her capacity as a leader. Beneath this need for leadership lie many dependency characteristics that have not been adequately fulfilled in her own childhood. A chronic repression of hostility is the most commonly encountered affect in our experience in response to the role requirements described above. This leads, in turn, to the clinical syndrome of reactive depression. The depression is reactive to the role stress and the relationship conflict in the marriage. This is frequently a chronic reactive syndrome. As we are dealing with a person with religious motivation, profound guilt feelings become a part of this clinical syndrome. The impulse is to strike out against the object or objects that deprive her. Because she cannot allow this in the context of her religious experience, she must internalize her feelings, and this results in a sense of "badness" and "unspirituality." Masochistic character traits are prominently present in this syndrome and sadomasochistic trends in the marriage add to the clinical complexity. Typically, these persons have a wish to hurt while allowing themselves to be chronically exposed to a process of being hurt. This has deep religious significance, because persecution is a religious expectation.

Other clinical manifestations as a result of the role stress are involved in a chronic sense of unfulfillment, particularly the crushing of youthful aspirations and ideals with the onset of middle age. At this point it often appears that the goal of the ministry has not been achieved as originally perceived. In addition, the turmoil the minister's wife witnesses in her own adolescent children reinforces

her sense of failure as a mother and as a wife. The deprivation of
sexual gratification, which previously she had been able to deny
as a consequence of her husband's chronic absence and her own
busy schedule, now becomes an acute problem. She may no longer
be able to hold back her sexual fantasy. She may project onto her
husband her own wish to establish relationships with others. This
often leads to a classic paranoid menopausal syndrome. At best,
the guilt it produces is disabling.

Middle age also brings with it for the minister's wife a profound
sense of insecurity. She is not allowed some of the traditional
sources of security of her peers. She does not have her own home,
but is dependent on the approval or disapproval of a congregation.
If her husband has not achieved professional prominence by his
middle forties, it is highly unlikely that he will later in life. There
is a financial stress to be faced in the future, with limited pension
fund, low income, and subservience to the gifts of the congregation.
These gifts, which were once seen as a boon, are now seen as
fickle. There seems to be a high incidence of psychosomatic disturbances in the minister's wife who comes for clinical attention. A
minister's wife, because of the guilt implied by being emotionally
ill, unconsciously seeks socially acceptable expressions of her emotional tension. Psychosomatic disorders often provide a shelter
tolerable to herself, her husband, and the congregation. We have
observed a large incidence of lower intestinal disturbances such as
spastic colitis. Headaches are also very common, and frequently
insight is fairly readily available into the dynamics of psychosomatic
disorders. Hostility is most often seen as the repressed affect.

Extensive clinical exposure to the problems of minister's children
as young children, adolescents, and college students, reveals several
typical syndromes. These children have come from backgrounds in
the United States and as missionary offspring. There is a typical
deprivation type syndrome of early age that leads to profound
adolescent turmoil and sometimes a psychotic decompensation.
Such children are at times hospitalized in late adolescence or young
adulthood with ego-diffusion and profound suicidal ideation. There

seems to be some truth in the observation that as the policeman's child needs to steal to express his rebellion against the family, so the minister's child needs to attack the bastion of Christian faith and hope because this is held so dear in the value system of the minister. This is particularly true of young persons in trouble on religious campuses. For the more neurotic child, who has incorporated much of the value structure of his society, compulsive defenses are needed to contain deviant impulses. There is a typical younger child that we refer to at this point, one who is noted for constriction and restriction of expression of emotional impulses, highly intellectualized and desexualized. Rather than a decompensatory break, this child, in later childhood or young adulthood, may face the inability to form heterosexual relationships, although he may be able to excel in intellectual pursuits. Despite the variety of theological persuasions among Protestant denominations, the mores have much in common. They tend to be restrictive and rigid, and they prepare children poorly for the adolescent period of growth and emotional experience. Since religious thinking tends to have an aura of nonproposition, that is, either it is sin or righteousness, the superego formation of these children tends to be very rigid and unyielding. One of the consequences of this is the formation of superego lacunae. Frequently, these children see in their parents an attempt to escape the rigid system; in a sense this gives them intuitive permission to find their own exceptions to the rule. Profound and very disturbing deviant behavior can result with little sense of guilt. Or, in contrast, there can be a profound sense of guilt for deviation from apparently relatively unimportant performance of religious rituals. Both reactions can be seen in the same young person. This thought-process split frequently characterizes adolescent schizophreniform illness. Adolescence has been a period of awe and concern for ministers and their wives and deeply religious persons in general because it is the period of life when the faith may die with the adolescent's rebellion against it. Strong inhibitions and restrictions have been built into the child's superego structure from an early age. This tends to produce adolescent rebellion of a very dramatic quality. If childhood deprivation, affect loss, and identification defects are present, this can result in an adolescent type of psychotic break.

TREATMENT

The treatment of the minister's wife can rarely be accomplished without her husband. This is a result of the fact that her concerns are concerns of the marriage and the family. To treat her foremost without providing her husband the opportunity for concurrent growth and for maturing in a marriage relationship is, in a sense, to place the marriage in greater jeopardy. The risk of psychotherapy in this context is that she may transcend her husband in insight and emotional capacities, which may profoundly disturb the marital balance. It is certainly true that there may be individual features in her background that must be explored as an individual. She may need to look at her motivation for becoming a minister's wife or her relationship to her own parents and her own emotional expectations up to the point of the marriage. However, she most typically will see her conflict in terms of the present relationships within the family and the relationship of her family to the congregation. She will deeply desire to have her husband present and will be resentful of him if he does not become a part of treatment. She will push for insight psychotherapy and not be satisfied with palliative measures such as the use of psychotropic drugs. The exception to this pattern would be the situation in which she has accepted the apparent fact that her husband will not look at the problem with her. She then may readily run for physiological relief from her symptoms. The minister's wife will typically form a very close treatment relationship with ease. This has its danger, as the dependency characteristics of therapy may become difficult to manage. The therapist of the minister's wife must beware of seductivity on her part and of her substituting the therapist for her husband. The apparent countertransference danger for the therapist arises from the ease with which he can sympathize with her plight. She may cast her husband in the role of the evil one and may insist that he make the ultimate sacrifice, namely, abandoning the ministry as his profession in order to retain a relationship with her. This is a particularly damaging threat, because separation and divorce or such dangerous alternatives within their religious structure have such great significance.

The treatment of the child of the minister is not usually possible without collaborative treatment of the parents in family therapy, depending on the clinical syndrome and the age of the child. In unusually severe cases, separation may be inevitable; it will be particularly difficult for the child to deal with because of his previous experience of deprivation through the work habits of the father. The child may be a conveyor and an expressor of the wife's hostility towards her husband's role and the attitudes of the church. The child's deviance may be her unconscious deviance. For the older child, the ability to verbalize his concerns and express emotional turmoil in direct terms is typically quite impossible. For the adolescent or young adult, an honest resolution of the relationship problems with the family must be part of treatment. Simple isolation or environmental manipulation of the problem is not usually adequate because of severe superego requirements. Psychotropic drugs usually have little value in these adolescent disturbances. Motivation for insight and working through the relationship problems is typically high. A confrontational type of resolution with the parents is highly desired by ministers' children. In fact, a crisis-type resolution is more typical in view of the religious background, with the characteristic expectation of religious conversion as a way of resolving problems. Both ministers' wives and children are gratifying patients because they typically bring with them a high degree of personal requirement for resolution of the problem. There is usually a sound structure to the personality and a stable value system within which the child is operating or against which he is reacting. They tend to seek clear resolutions rather than simply move from one shade of gray to another.

SUMMARY

Clinical research in the understanding of psychotherapy of the minister's wife and children is desperately needed [6]. This can best be done against the background of specific cultural understandings. It would be impossible to perceive the clinical syndromes without understanding the value structure and role stresses that have been described above.

REFERENCES

1. Denton, W. *The Role of the Minister's Wife*. Philadelphia: Westminster Press, 1962.
2. Denton, W. *The Minister's Wife as a Counselor*. Philadelphia: Westminster Press, 1965.
3. Douglas, W. *Ministers' Wives*. New York: Harper and Row, 1965.
4. Hartman, O. *The Holy Masquerade*. Grand Rapids, Mich.: W. B. Eerdmans, 1963.
5. Oden, M. B. *The Minister's Wife: A Person or Position*. New York: Abingdon, 1966.
6. Pattison, E. Social and psychological aspects of religion in psychotherapy. *J. Nerv. Ment. Dis.* 141:586, 1966.
7. Smith, C. *How to Become a Bishop Without Being Religious*. New York: Doubleday, 1965.

The Mental Health of Members of Religious Communities

ROBERT J. MC ALLISTER

INTRODUCTION

A segment of popular opinion, which is not at all limited to the irreligious, considers the person who enters a religious community as definitely peculiar. The basic premise to support this opinion seems to be that the life of a religious is an abnormal kind of existence. The vows or promises that religious take and that involve the areas of obedience, chastity, and poverty are considered to be an unnatural abrogation of certain basic tendencies and a frustration of fundamental needs. Even the modified or temporary forms of these three vows, which are becoming increasingly popular in religious communities, are unacceptable to critics of religious life. Those who take these vows, even without the element of permanency, are adjudged eccentric, if not irrational.

PUBLISHED STUDIES AND RESULTS

Probably because of this popular suspicion that religious life and mental illness must be highly correlated, two outstanding studies of the incidence of mental illness in Catholic religious have been conducted. It is noteworthy that both studies have been conducted by Catholic religious. Reverend Thomas Verner Moore [4] published an article in the *American Ecclesiastical Review* in 1936 entitled, "Insanity in Priests and Religious." His work was essentially a comparison of the incidence of mental illness among Catholic priests and religious in the United States with the incidence of mental illness in the country's general population. Moore concluded that mental illness occurred more frequently among the general population than among the religious on a per capita basis. He noted a significantly higher rate of mental illness among cloistered nuns as opposed to non-cloistered.

Sister Mary William Kelley [1] in her 1958 article in the *American Journal of Psychiatry,* concluded that mental illness among sisters was increasing more rapidly than it was in the general population of women in the United States, although the incidence of mental illness was still considerably lower among religious women.

A later series of studies by McAllister and VanderVeldt [2, 3, 5] makes some conclusions that may account in part for the results obtained by Moore and Kelley. McAllister and VanderVeldt compared data from the records of 100 priests and 100 nuns hospitalized for mental illness, selected by consecutive discharge dates, and data from the records of 100 male patients and 100 female patients consecutively discharged from the same mental hospital. It was found that religious patients had diagnoses of personality disorders twice as often as lay patients. The reverse was true in the diagnostic categories of affective and involutional psychoses and psychoneurotic depressive reactions. The incidence of organic brain syndromes and of schizophrenic reactions was approximately the same in the religious and lay populations. These data suggest that the symptomatology of mental illness may differ for the two groups. There is the further implication that the kind of mental illness to which religious are susceptible may only require hospitalization in a small percentage of cases. Personality disorders in the hospital may represent a small segment of the number outside the hospital. On the other hand, affective and involutional psychoses and psychoneurotic depressive reactions represent potential suicide and are usually quickly hospitalized by treating physicians.

There has been substantial resistance in most religious communities to psychiatric care for community members. It is possible that the kind of psychopathology in religious communities does not vary from the psychopathology among lay groups as much as the reaction in the environment varies. Religious communities tolerate very poorly the deviant member whose acting-out behavior may be the result of a sociopathic personality structure. The same community may, on the other hand, show little concern for the chronically depressed, rather withdrawn member whose symptoms might stimulate a psychiatrist to recommend hospitalization. There is a kind of myth that counteracts the average person's, and especially the physician's, concern for the religious who is depressed. The myth is that a deeply religious person would not commit suicide. An active faith in religious principles gives meaning and value to one's existence. When one's mood is so dejected as to dull the force of one's faith, the emotional loss that ensues may increase the depth of despondency.

EMOTIONAL STRESS IN RELIGIOUS LIFE

Life in a religious community has its own particular stresses. The vows that are made and the limitations that these impose are, in a sense, stressful situations. Obedience is undoubtedly a source of greater emotional conflict than the vow of chastity is. Obedience to the authority of a superior is never easy for an adult to attain. Lack of maturity in the adult makes the attainment of a proper attitude toward authority a virtual impossibility. The psychology of religious life has many parallels with the psychology of adolescence. Both states make demands on the individual to act like an adult, but place him in the role of the dependent child. The religious depends on his superiors, not just for his position, not just for his livelihood, but for the tenor of his very existence. This is a constant relationship that pervades all corners of the subject's life and permeates his day-to-day living in myriad subtle manners.

The very intensity of this interrelationship precipitates the religious subject into the probability of transference phenomena that may never be resolved. Caught up in conflicts that should have been resolved when he matured from adolescence to adulthood, the religious distorts his own relationship with his superior and converts the spirit of obedience into a sort of servitude. It is typical of this condition among members of religious communities as well as among adolescents that they perceive the authority figure as the one who needs to change in order to establish a harmonious interrelationship. Their introspective ability is considerably limited.

The position of dependency in which the religious subject is placed severely limits the range of his negative reactions to his superiors. It is difficult to allow oneself to express anger toward those on whom one depends a great deal. Angry feelings become a threat to oneself in such a situation. It becomes necessary to curtail their expression in fear of possible retaliation on the part of the omnipotent authority figure. Various psychological problems can result from the overcontrol of anger. The frequency of psychosomatic illness among religious has a close relationship with the unexpressed anger frequently present in their lives.

It is evident that obedience creates a dual difficulty for members of religious communities. First, it places the religious in a dependent position that involves many aspects of his life. Second, it prevents him from reacting to the frustration of that very relationship.

The vow of celibacy also has a twofold meaning for members of religious communities. There is the obvious prohibition against sexual satisfaction per se. This is difficult enough for the average religious, whose natural desires in this regard are normal in intensity. There is also considerable conflict created for the religious who finds it difficult to distinguish between sexual and sensual in the broader sense of the latter term. Confusion in the interpretation of sensual pleasures can make them appear illicit, when they are in no way so. If there is such confusion, the religious may deprive himself of many normal and healthy outlets for physical tension and emotional fatigue.

The confusion of sexual pleasures with feelings of affection creates additional conflicts for many religious. They may deprive themselves of proper satisfactions that are vital for human happiness, because they adhere so sanctimoniously to their false interpretation of a virtue. Their need to love and their need to be loved are not altered by the taking of a vow. Their expression of these needs must, however, be modified. To participate in human love should not be considered impossible to them nor inappropriate for their way of life.

THE PROBLEM OF IDENTITY IN THE RELIGIOUS

One of the factors that has received much attention in the psychology of the religious life is the problem of identity. Present-day society has become preoccupied with this problem as a result of several cultural trends, one of which revolves around the "new breed" in religious life. The young religious is searching for his identity. Though his quest is often excused on the basis of youth, there seems to be a marked trend upward in the chronological age of those who need to find themselves. It is unfortunate for the future of religious communities that so many of their members have a need to work out these basic confusions after they become active and often influential community members. The stability of any institution or organization must be disturbed by the instability of numerous important members. Such members are quite sharply identified within the community. The result is that the community identifies them clearly and conspicuously, thus making their personal lack of identification so much more egregious.

Some greater development of a sense of identity prior to entering the religious community or in the preliminary phases of the commitment is very much in order. The enthusiasm and vitality of youth, identified or not, are an asset to any organization or group. If these same youth control the colleges and universities, there will cease to be colleges and universities as they presently exist. If these same youth take over political power, the government as it is and functions will no longer be. If these same youth are allowed to direct the structure and spirit of religious communities, if they are permitted to change those communities to fit themselves instead of changing themselves to fit the communities, then religious communities in their present form will be brought to an end.

The need to establish one's own identity, the importance of knowing who one is within oneself and in relation to the world outside, is obviously of prime importance in individual psychology. To arrive at this significant knowledge, one must have a stabile system of external values and independent criteria. If the external environment is distorted in an attempt to achieve one's own identity, the end product of this effort must necessarily be inaccurate. There are many contemporary religious who are trying to change their community and their church in a vain endeavor to make themselves identifiable in the institution they might then create. This religious will be no more content in the new order than he was in the old, because he will not yet have achieved an independent identity. The reformer is more likely to be more understanding with problems and more successful with answers if he establishes first his own identity, then his community membership, and finally his position as a proponent of renewal of what is worthwhile and reform of what is unsatisfactory.

There is a special kind of identity problem that seems peculiarly inherent in the religious life. There is such a complete dedication required of the religious that he nearly loses his own identity in the process. There is no comparable life role in which the individual must be so totally occupied. The religious is a religious 24 hours a day, 365 days a year. In the classroom, on the street, on vacation, in private quarters, he is always a religious and is expected to behave in certain ways because of that fact. There is an inescapable burden in such a role. There is an inevitable hazard. The religious can lose his personal identity through an overidentification with his religious role. He becomes more concerned about himself as a religious than as a human being. He loses sight of the fact that his basic worth depends on his human nature rather than on his superimposed religious character. Such an attitude creates conflict with others who may be less deceived by his religious role than he is. Such an attitude creates conflict within the individual, because it ties his basic worth to a secondary function. It is then so easy to become an aggressive religious, an omnipotent religious, a sanctimonious religious, because one's worth, one's identity is hinged to that role.

EFFECT OF FAMILY BACKGROUND

It is probable that some individuals who enter the religious life have a predisposition to mental illness. It is possible that certain personality traits that contributed to this choice of life may also contribute to mental disturbance. The home environment from which an individual comes certainly contributes to his choice of role in adult life. It is not unusual to find that a religious has come from a rather strict home, which was prayer-oriented and sometimes ceremoniously organized. A parental interpretation of the Ten Commandments may have been used as the proximate norm of conduct. Emotional expression may have been somewhat stilted, with definite parental dissuasion regarding any manifestation of anger and absolute ignoring of the existence of sexuality in the world. Hostile expressions by children were contrary to the Fourth Commandment and required repentance. Sexual interest was not dealt with directly but only brushed aside, unseen.

The articles by McAllister and VanderVeldt suggest a connection between mental pathology in religious and their relationships with their parents. The typical picture among mentally ill religious was a closeness to the parent of the opposite sex. This relationship occurred significantly more often among religious patients than among lay patients. Of the 100 mentally ill clergy studied, 91% came from homes in which the mother was the dominant figure and 86% came from homes in which one parent exhibited definite psychiatric symptoms, frequently alcoholism on the part of the father [2].

It is quite possible that the two factors just mentioned, i.e., closeness to the parent of the opposite sex and psychopathology in the home, contribute to the choice of religious life as well as to the emotional problems of some religious. Identification with the parent of the opposite sex and consequent sexual confusion may be resolved in part by choosing a life of celibacy. For some, the resolution is not adequate, and subsequent sexual pathology is the result. Of the 100 clergymen involved in the study previously quoted, 38 had symptomatology in the sexual area (unpublished material). Sexual symptoms for purposes of that study would be defined as sexual behavior that obviously deviated from chosen goals and created problems for the individuals exhibiting the behavior.

The article on alcoholism in clergymen [5] sketches the "most likely portrait of the alcoholic priest" and includes the following reference to family background: "His mother was the dominant figure in the home, and he was closer to her, although he identified with the weaker, frequently alcoholic father. There is a good possibility that he was the oldest child or the only boy in the family."

EFFECT OF SEMINARY TRAINING

The religiously oriented, strict home life, in which independent thought and behavior is stifled, produces an individual who is psychologically suited to the successful completion of religious training. This is true because the training environment for the religious candidate is a duplication of that kind of environment. Consequently, the candidate from such a background adjusts most easily to the training phase of religious life. Since that training phase is intended to be a testing phase as well, this particular candidate is naturally prepared to complete the period without difficulty.

It is this same individual who may then find the transition from seminary to service a most difficult one. Of the 200 religious patients involved in the above study [3], 97 had the onset of psychiatric symptoms before age 33. Seventy of the lay group had psychiatric symptoms prior to that age. Nearly one-half of the group of religious patients were emotionally ill prior to or within five years of their entrance into active religious life following the initial training period.

The religious candidate who has had the questionable security of a strict home life and the immaturity of a background emotionally dampened by scrupulous spirituality has not been forced to progress to a level of independence and maturity during the period of his novitiate. The adjustment requirements as he enters the nonprotective world of everyday living are often greater than his coping mechanism can bear. One result is psychiatric illness. Another is frank defection from religious life or the partial defection of those who remain but temper their service with selfishness. Another result is the desperate attempt to force authority figures to maintain their protective jurisdiction by presenting them with attitudinal and behavior patterns that stimulate the desired response.

COMMON PSYCHIATRIC PROBLEMS

Some of the more common psychiatric syndromes among religious are the result of this discrepancy between the need to be mature as an active religious in an adult world and the inability to do so because of inadequate personality development in early life and inappropriate psychological stimulation during the training process. The study of priests [2] that has been mentioned found 15 sociopaths among the group of 100, an unusually high ratio. Forty-six of the 100 clergy had a diagnosis of personality disorder. The sexual and alcoholic acting-out behavior that is typical of this group is a kind of partial defection, which provides the continued social and financial security of community affiliation.

It is a rather striking statistic that nearly one-half of the hospitalized clergy were diagnosed as personality disorders. The religious women in the study [3] showed a high proportion of personality disorders, especially of the paranoid and schizoid type. Personality disorders among the 200 religious patients were twice as frequent as among the 200 lay patients. "Perhaps it is in religious life that the individual with a personality disorder achieves some comfort. Close interpersonal relationships are generally discouraged, so their ineptness in this regard is not strained. On the other hand, the irritation and discord which these individuals frequently arouse in others are diluted by the Christian charity practiced by their associates." [3]

Among religious women, the clinical syndrome that most frequently comes to the attention of the psychiatrist could be classified as a paranoid personality disturbance. This patient considers her superiors as basically in error in their management of her problems. She sometimes, at least on a verbal level, gives them credit for trying, but carefully delineates their obvious failures. Not only the superior, but the community, does not understand her, and there is patent injustice in this attitude. There is little hope on the part of the patient that a genuine understanding and meeting of the minds with her superior can ever be accomplished. She is probably more accurate in this conclusion than her superiors, who spend an undue portion of their time and energy in attempting to help her.

The incidence of alcoholism is rare among religious women, undoubtedly because of the obvious difficulties in obtaining regular supplies. With increasing freedom to move about in less conspicuous attire, it is likely that the incidence will increase. Proneness to become habituated is present among women in religious communities. This propensity has been satisfied by the abuse of drugs, particularly of the amphetamine and barbiturate groups. Their personal physicians would often find it difficult to believe that someone in religious life would be interested in some method of pharmacological relief. Consequently, they may write prescription after prescription without the element of suspicion to provide them with caution.

FACTORS IN TREATMENT

Just as the average physician has confidence in the emotional stability and personal honesty of the individual religious, so the psychiatrist may be misled by his own parataxic distortions regarding "the religious." The examining doctor, whether he be a psychiatrist or not, tends to see the religious patient in that guise of "religious" and has difficulty looking beneath this superficial role to the human being, who assimilates food, who breathes, who gets angry, who needs security the same as other human beings do. The religious patient in psychotherapy has a natural tendency to protect himself by the use of his religious role. He philosophizes about himself easily, but he discusses his true feelings with great difficulty. He will discuss love of God and of neighbor in preference to talking about his own anger or his own sensual attraction to another human being. This is his protective mechanism, which he employs for his own psychological equilibrium, which he displays to the credulous world, and which he applies to the therapeutic endeavor to resist the discomfort of change.

This countertransference, to which the therapist is so vulnerable, and this conscious, or more likely unconscious, subterfuge on the part of the religious patient are not the only handicaps in the psychiatric care of religious. The general attitude of religious superiors toward psychiatric evaluation and care has been a strongly negative one. Attacks on the profession of psychiatry by prominent members of the hierarchy have done much to maintain a distrustful and misinformed attitude on the part of religious communities toward the appropriate use of psychiatric consultation and treatment.

Fortunately, a great deal is being done to alleviate this shallow attitude on the part of religious. The Academy of Religion and Mental Health has pioneered a great deal of this effort. Mental health workshops for clergymen and for members of religious communities for women have made an outstanding contribution to increased understanding of the role of psychiatry in improving the emotional health of individual religious and of religious communities. The Pastoral Workshop at St. John's University in Collegeville, Minnesota, is the oldest and most eminent of these workshops.

Most people share the difficulty of distinguishing between deviant behavior that is the result of a mental problem and deviant behavior that is a deliberate defiance of rules, social codes, natural ethics, or divine law. Among the members of religious communities, deviant behavior is more likely evaluated as resulting from a lack of sanctity rather than from a lack of sanity. The religious who seeks psychiatric help often views himself and is viewed by his confreres as a failure in the religious life. This attitude makes it difficult to seek psychiatric care in the early phase of illness. The life of the religious has its own peculiar stresses, its own particular problems. It is unfortunate that psychiatric care, which can be a source of equilibrium and satisfaction, should become instead a source of anxiety and guilt.

REFERENCES

1. Kelley, M. W. The incidence of hospitalized mental illness among religious sisters in the U.S. *Amer. J. Psychiat.* 115:72, 1958.
2. McAllister, R. J., and VanderVeldt, A. J. Factors in mental illness among hospitalized clergy. *J. Nerv. Ment. Dis.* 132:80, 1961.
3. McAllister, R. J., and VanderVeldt, A. J. Psychiatric illness in hospitalized Catholic religious. *Amer. J. Psychiat.* 121:881, 1965.
4. Moore, T. V. Insanity in priests and religious. *Amer. Ecclesiast. Rev.* 95:485 and 95:601, 1936.
5. VanderVeldt, A. J., and McAllister, R. J. Psychiatric illness in hospitalized clergy: Alcoholism. *Quart. J. Stud. Alcohol.* 23:124, 1962.

Evaluating Candidates for Religious Service

RICHARD H. COX AND TRUMAN G. ESAU

CANDIDATE EVALUATION

In recent years, increasing attention has been given to the psychodynamic evaluation of persons for religious service. The early pioneer evaluators received very little training except to establish the orthodoxy of their doctrine. However, quite early in the history of candidate evaluation, attention was given to soundness of body. Candidates were examined for physical fitness, but little or no thought was given to psychic and interpersonal functioning. To question one's emotional health was tantamount to doubting one's faith. It was assumed that religious personnel did not have psychological problems.

Historically, the innovation of psychosomatic medicine brought with it the necessity of taking a closer look at the "physical" ailments of religious personnel, particularly returnees. This new emphasis in holistic medicine pointed out the relationship between psychological tension and physical disease. It was soon learned that a significant number of returnees were suffering from psychological problems that often precipitated or exacerbated organic difficulties. It was at that point that mental health personnel became involved. Vocational testing, personality assessment, and "screening" began to play an important part in the candidate selection.

Today, more and more missionary boards, religious orders, and other appointing bodies are requiring psychological and psychiatric evaluation. Although few, if any, of these groups would appoint a candidate with disabling organic pathology, often persons have been appointed with serious neurotic or psychotic tendencies. These persons not only possess the germs for their own psychological disease, but they have the potential for contributing to interpersonal conflict.

It is assumed that mental health consultants will be of the highest certification available in their respective professional disciplines. However, traditional training in these disciplines does not of itself prepare the evaluator to understand the cultural and emotional involvement of this specialized group of persons. This will only come with the experience of such evaluations and the intimate interaction with the appointing bodies of the groups under discussion. The evaluator must be aware of the value systems implicit and explicit in the candidates. He must be aware of his own value systems, against which he judges the candidates.

Traditional evaluation of the intrapsychic mechanisms of an individual candidate, as important as it may be, has not proved to be adequate for the task of evaluating candidates for religious service. These techniques were adequate to identify definable psychic pathology, but they have not been sufficient to provide the appointing board with an integrated view of the person's intrapsychic structure, interpersonal transactions, and social adaptability. The training and experience of several different mental health professions have been utilized in this task. Appointing bodies have referred their candidates to clinical psychologists for evaluation by the use of established psychological tools. The psychologist might have been asked to make the clinical evaluation at the same time. Or the candidate has been sent to an individual psychiatrist for the clinical evaluation, supplemented by psychological evaluation by a clinical psychologist, not necessarily in the same geographic vicinity. A gap that has resulted from these practices is the lack of coordination of the efforts of these professional opinions. As a consequence, an appointing body would have highly technical reports, which were difficult for them to coordinate, or the professional could feel it necessary to give only a brief summary statement, which did not give sufficient data upon which to act. It has been typical for examiners, utilizing this approach, to appraise psychic pathology primarily, and fail to evaluate the balance of assets and disabilities in the candidates' emotional construction. This does not meet the needs of the referring religious agencies. This is particularly true since most candidates do not show a traditional frank psychiatric disorder.

Certain obvious handicaps arise from utilizing professions in a fragmented manner. It can be stated that the least effective professional evaluation of a candidate is that which is done by a practitioner, a clinical psychologist, or a psychiatrist who is relatively unacquainted with the group for whom he is doing the evaluation and who only sees the candidate for one interview. If the examiner is not related through the process of working out professional ties with the religious group, he will tend to see the candidate only in the terms of his own professional stereotypes. Furthermore, he will be handicapped in the utilization of his material, for he will not be aware of the use to which the referring group will put it.

A more valuable approach is one utilizing the skills of both the clinical psychologist and the psychiatrist. It has been typical to utilize two such professionals, but often with little collaboration. This has been a product of geographical limitations and financial concerns.

A clinical psychologist and a psychiatrist, functioning as a work team, offer an improved medium for accomplishing the goal of evaluation. This is a product of their ability to collaborate as well as of their emotional cathexis to one another as a result of shared practice. The best clinical tool available at this time is that of a multidisciplinary team, which should include the psychiatric social worker as well as a clinical psychologist and psychiatrist. The insights of the anthropologist or sociologist would be a great asset, but realistically they are not available for such collaboration at the present time.

A psychiatric social history designed to meet the needs of candidate evaluation will be characterized by a longitudinal descriptive picture of the life history of the candidate. This will include material regarding the candidate's early growth and development, family relationships, educational achievements, and development of motivation for religious service, and appraisals of how the candidate has coped with past stress and of the candidate's ability to form meaningful, healthy interpersonal relationships. An adequate history will extend beyond the normal to include deviant and pathological maladaptations and medical and psychiatric illness. It will aid in an overall holistic integration of psychosocial data.

Adequate psychodiagnostic testing will include pencil-and-paper evaluations, such as the Minnesota Multiphasic Personality Inventory, the California Psychological Inventory, and other well-validated measures of health and pathology. It will also include the projective techniques, such as the Rorschach Psychodiagnostic Test and the Thematic Apperception Test, which allow an evaluation of the unconscious dynamics at work. The testing will also include other specific tests as thought necessary by the examiner [5].

The psychiatric evaluation will screen the candidate for gross psychiatric pathology. It will confirm the presence of adequate reality testing or identify gross defects in this process. In addition, there will be an assessment of ego functioning from which an evaluation of the defense mechanisms utilized by this individual in the handling of stress can be made. There will be a measure from the clinical interview of the capacity of the individual to form interpersonal relationships and even to cope with the stress implicit in the interview itself. This interview may not only assess the individual dynamics, but may also evaluate the dynamics of the marital situation if the candidate is being evaluated with his spouse.

Evaluating personnel for any occupation is difficult, but it is complicated beyond words when there is no job description. What are the personality traits of a "good" candidate for religious service? Are they the same as for any other successful person? Do different geographic locations demand more or less of a given personality? It is imperative that religious bodies seeking candidate evaluation supply the evaluator with as adequate a job description as possible. References have been found to be notoriously superficial and obviously given by persons whom the candidate felt would supply an optimistic view of his capabilities.

The crucial factor involved in team appraisal is the integration of the data into a meaningful gestalt. Let us first consider the candidate who will be approved and whose functioning would be considered within the normal range. The referring religious body desires and deserves more than this simple statement. It is interested in knowing the assets and liabilities of a given candidate in respect to a specific geographical locale and job description. Traditional "screening out" is not sufficient, for there is as yet no valid research that identifies precisely enough those who should be screened out. Except for gross psychiatric pathology, it is presumptive for the mental health practitioner to assume this level of judgment. Therefore, an overall mental health portrait is given to the referring body, which aids the group in deciding if that particular kind of personality can be utilized. This portrait will include perceptive statements about the candidate's intrapsychic adjustment, i.e., the inner resources of the person's emotional, intellectual, and motivational acumen. It will include illustrative data regarding past and present interpersonal adjustments and predictive statements regarding future adjustments. Since any given candidate will not function equally well in every situation, it is imperative that the referring agency be cognizant of the candidate's capacity for leadership, his relationship to authority, and his ability to assume responsibility, and that it be given a frank appraisal of the candidate's sexual adjustment in marriage or sublimation-type activities [2, 7, 8].

PATHOLOGY

There are some typical clinical syndromes that are readily observable in the course of routine evaluation of candidates for religious service. The mental health observer is in no position to assume that strong religious motivation of itself is necessarily pathological. However, there are some typical clinical syndromes that are only observable by the mental health examiner. Considerable clinical research is necessary to determine whether or not a candidate who is willing to deviate from sociocultural norms is psychopathological or psychologically healthy. This is intimately tied up with the value systems implicit in the religious structure and their utilization by the individual candidate. The person's need hierarchy is the base for which he perceives the requirements of the service to which he is applying. These requirements include sexual, social, financial, and other sacrifices. The referring body will be looking to the practitioner for insight into the possible existence of psychologically unsound motivations and characterological formations in the candidate, which will identify those candidates who handle the value systems of the culture in a pathological fashion. The examiner will become aware of certain patterns that typify given religious bodies. Through intensive contact with these groups, he will come to see how these syndromes function pathologically in the areas of religious service and will help to identify them, either for rejection as candidates or for specialized placement in areas where their pathology will do a minimum amount of damage to their peers or to the persons to whom they minister, and where their assets will be most utilized.

Even in the identification of frank psychiatric disorders, such as persistent characterological defects, psychotic disturbances, and the more classic neurotic manifestations, it must be remembered that religious persons will tend to express their symptoms through religious ideation. This will make them difficult to identify, for the examiner must differentiate between the religious ideology per se and its use as a psychological defense. This is particularly true in the preparanoid states. Compulsivity, depressive tendencies, and passive-dependent mechanisms also frequently appear under the guise of religious observance. In our experience, the most frequent syndrome for the expression of many of the psychiatric disorders in Protestant missionary candidates is the pathological inability to form and maintain significant intimate interpersonal relationships. Religious rigidity is a phenomenon frequently observed in such persons, accompanied by pathological guilt feelings. The norm expected of these religious leaders is to handle their problems through religious observance, such as prayer, study of the Scripture, and sacraments, without reference to in-depth understanding of their own functioning as persons [6, 9].

PROJECTED NEEDS

The evaluation of religious personnel is going to demand increased involvement of social science and mental health specialists. Preventive planning in all phases will become more important. The following are only a few of our speculations. Some of them are now being done in part by some religious bodies.

Detailed field studies, utilizing anthropologists, sociologists, psychologists, and other specialists, will be necessary to arrive at adequate job descriptions, training requirements, and personality factors needed. These factors will vary with geographic locale. For instance, a candidate who is able to adjust to Oriental culture may not be able to make an adequate adjustment in Brazil. Many emotional problems are precipitated in part by cultural expectations and inabilities to adapt to them. There are persons and marriages that will remain essentially healthy in Western culture, with its stresses, but that cannot adjust to a different society and its expectations. Before proper preparation can be made, more and more of these factors must be known.

Family evaluations must be made. It is not enough to examine the candidate. Even bodies that consider the male spouse to be the primary candidate readily recognize that his wife's assets and liabilities will affect the overall work [1]. Many of these bodies now evaluate both the husband and the wife, but few evaluate the children. The children are subjected to boarding school, home teaching, and a variety of other conditions with very limited knowledge of their intellectual, academic, and emotional potential. What happens to the slow learner, the poor reader, or the retarded? What happens to the potential of the gifted child? Why should we assume that all children are able to adjust to life away from parents for many months at a time? What happens to children with physical and emotional handicaps? Perhaps at least a partial answer for the planning for children of religious personnel may be found in thorough studies of the children prior to their overseas placement, and subsequent evaluation on furloughs for follow-up and for children who have been born overseas [3, 4].

Required orientation programs for candidates are helpful to integrate their specialized training with the expectations of religious mission. Specialized training does not necessarily equip one for the given task of religious service to which he has been appointed.

Required personal counseling would be invaluable as a preventive measure. The person who knows his strengths and weaknesses is in a far better position to cope with pressure and change. At the present time, most organizations secure psychological evaluation but utilize the results only for consultative purposes. Some allow for an additional conference with the examiner for personal interpretation. These results would be far more valuable if they could be used for both consultative and counseling purposes.

Reevaluation at each furlough is important. Many changes occur in one's life and thinking within a term of service. In addition, the candidate, due to a rapidly changing world scene, often must be sent to a different field than the one for which he was originally evaluated. Previous psychological-psychiatric material should be made available for such reexaminations. Comparative studies are important when viewing the process of personality change.

SUMMARY

The psychodiagnostic evaluation of candidates for religious service is a specialized task. It should include more than the exclusion of gross pathology, and should optimally provide guidelines on where and how a candidate may be expected to function effectively or experience difficulties. Knowledge of the value systems of the religious organization and knowledge of the potential field of service are essential for providing meaningful evaluations. Greater attention must be given to a candidate's spouse and family in making evaluations, and greater consideration to preventive measures, including orientation and counseling, is currently needed.

REFERENCES

1. Ackerman, N. *The Psychodynamics of Family Life*. New York: Basic Books, 1958.
2. Arnold, M. B., Hispanicus, P., Weisgerber, C. A., and D'Arcy, P. F. *Screening Candidates for the Priesthood and Religious Life*. Chicago: Loyola University Press, 1962.
3. Bailey, H. L., and Jackson, H. C. *A Study of Missionary Motivation, Training, and Withdrawal (1953–1962)*. New York: Missionary Research Library, 1965.
4. Bakwin, H., and Bakwin, R. *Clinical Management of Behavior Disorders in Children*. Philadelphia: Saunders, 1960.
5. Horrocks, J. *Assessment of Behavior*. Columbus, Ohio: Charles E. Hall, 1964.
6. Oates, W. E. *Religious Factors in Mental Illness*. New York: Association Press, 1955.
7. Rosengrant, J. (Ed.). *Assignment: Overseas*. New York: Thomas Y. Crowell, 1966.
8. Torre, M. (Ed.). *The Selection of Personnel for International Service*. New York: World Federation for Mental Health, 1963.
9. VanderVeldt, J. H., and Odenwald, R. P. *Psychiatry and Catholicism*. New York: McGraw-Hill, 1952.

Psychotherapy of Religious Conflict*

MARGARETTA K. BOWERS

Although the lawful properties of personality development are still under dispute within and outside psychoanalytic thought, there is almost no disagreement on the fundamental role of conflict in healthy and sick development. Psychological health is promoted by effective solutions to conflict, solutions that permit expression and gratification of needs without grossly offending social and personal ethics. Conversely, psychogenic symptoms, character disorders, and psychoses are primarily promoted and maintained by ineffective solutions to conflict, solutions that stifle the expression of need or fail to integrate such expression into an appropriate social context.

In addition to the principle that conflict lies at the base of almost all psychogenic maladjustment, there is one more fundamental concept that must be interwoven for more complete understandings: This principle asserts that the degree of maladjustment stemming from a conflict is directly related to the extent to which the conflicting material is conscious; the more deeply buried the conflict, or any part of it, the greater the likelihood of severe symptom development.

It is this human ability to bury raw conflict under piles of defenses of intellect, affect, and somatic change that gives rise to the first hurdle in psychotherapy—the uncovering and isolating of the

* Grateful acknowledgement is given to Thea Spyer, Ph.D., for her creative editorial assistance in the preparation of this paper.

conflict for both therapist and patient. If this is true of all humans, why then a paper on psychotherapy of religious conflict or of conflict peculiar to the religiously concerned? There is admittedly no conflict or set of conflicts that are entirely peculiar to the religious. These persons suffer from the basic conflicts around such dimensions as sex, aggression, and dependency, and they also embrace the uncanny human ability to symbolize these conflicts in seemingly unrelated spheres of life. What is unique to this group is their having available a series of ideas, constructs, symbols, and rituals through which they strive for a philosophy and way of being but through which also they tend to experience and express their own fundamental humanness, which includes conflicts of many sorts. To paraphrase for emphasis, it must be understood that the ideas and acts of the devout serve to facilitate the creation and expression of a deeply meaningful order in existence and that these very same ideas, symbols, and acts can become distorted to serve as carriers of deep psychological problems and pathological solutions.

In the psychotherapy of the patient who comes with religious problems, the therapist has two great goals. One is the generally understood goal of helping the patient work through fixations, regressions, and those forms of insufficient development that give rise to religion and to nonreligious symptoms.

Second, it is the duty of the therapist to help the patient find a good religion and God-idea that permits and encourages personality growth and maturity.

In order to facilitate the patient's achieving the second goal, the therapist must know to view the ideation of religion as he does ideation of music or poetry. Common to all these fields is the special kind of reality that we attribute to an idea—to a way of looking at and manipulating the hard data of our own needs and our environment.

It thus becomes obvious that if the therapist wants to do good therapy with these people, there must be a therapeutic climate of acceptance of religion and devotion as a fact of life [7, 8].

The therapist may or may not be devout. If he is devout, his own personal religion should have had sufficient personal analysis, so that he is not hampered by blind spots caused by his own unconscious conflicts, and he should have had sufficient supervision of his work with religious conflicts to show that the conflicts he may have had are worked through.

If the therapist is not devout, his personal analysis and supervision should be of sufficient depth to make sure that he has not denied religious conflict but just was not deeply indoctrinated in religion as a child and adolescent. Such a therapist hopefully should have good "inner resources," and have the empathy to respect the patient's devotion just as he would respect his patient's creativity in any of the arts. He can understand a good religious vocation, as he can a vocation to be a poet; both are poorly paid as a rule, but as the creative person has to be creative to remain or become healthy, so the creativity of the devout has to be equally used.

The fact of God's existence in outer reality cannot be demonstrated, and should not be challenged, except to rid the God-idea of all human transference attitudes.

If the therapist is a good amateur anthropologist, he will have less of a problem coping with all the numerous faiths and denominations in our culture. Whenever he feels that a doctrine or God-idea is psychologically pathogenic, he should himself seek theological consultation. Sending the patient to find theological help may leave the patient in the same conflict. Patients have an uncanny ability to find pastors and confessors to reinforce their pathology, so that more harm than good may result unless the patient is sent to a good and wise theologian or a good and wise confessor. The therapist should question the soundness of the theology of any theologian who expounds a pathogenic doctrine and should seek further and more learned consultation. He must always remember that what is required dogma in one faith or denomination is not always exactly the same in another. Most denominations accept a symbolic interpretation of creed and doctrine, yet some of the fundamentalist members of the same denomination (both Catholic and Protestant) insist on the literal meaning of the same doctrine.

Religious doctrine is a question not of historical fact but of emotional need [9]. The language of religion is primary-process picture-language thinking and feeling. Resurrection is the feeling that "God has always been with me," and so in death, "He will still be with me—I am not alone, and He will not abandon me." [2, 7]

Armed with the flexibility to move comfortably among levels of experience, including the religious, the psychotherapist or psychoanalyst is prepared to explore religious conflict in its varied manifestations.

Conflict may come about on the very simple level of lack of intellectual adult religious education in the mature religious theology of one's denomination. A person who has been permitted or encouraged to think and learn mature concepts of science and evolution develops feelings of guilt and rebellion due to the continued effort to live within the theology he was taught as a child [3].

Thirty years ago, evolution was heresy in denominations that today explain that just as Jesus spoke in parables in the New Testament, so God spoke in parables in the Old Testament. There are practically no denominations that an intelligent, well-educated person would have difficulty with if he knew the mature concepts of his denomination and had the maturity to be tolerant of the immature attitudes of many members and clergy of his congregation. The mature adult can live with conscious conflict. Many Roman Catholics have been able to use contraception without guilt, accepting it as a small sin in the eyes of the Church, but with a deep sense of conviction that in time the attitude of the Church would change just as it did in relation to astronomy in the past.

Another clue to religious conflict is in the person who has converted from one denomination to another of radically different theology. The old religion is repressed on a childhood level of understanding but remains operative and distorts the new and more liberal theology to which the convert has turned.

This also can occur within the same denomination as a failure of integration of the childhood religion, which is, instead, repressed but operative. This most frequently occurs when the repression is the result of severe trauma, such as the death of a parent or sibling, before the age of five years [2, 5, 6]. Even the memory of such a death may be repressed. This can also occur at any age if the trauma is severe and the patient vulnerable.

One of the most important concepts in tracing and relating the presence of symptom-producing repressed ideation about the parents of patients in religion conflict may be referred to as God-transference. The God-idea occurs as a transference of the emotional reaction of and to the parents. The patient seems to have skipped over the more customary transference to therapist, social authorities, or fellow group members and instead acts out the fundamental transference from the parents directly upon the God-idea. In order to reach the emotions of this transference and slowly pull them back, as it were, to the original object, the therapist must analyze directly in the transference to the God-idea. Having isolated the transferred material as it is manifested in the God-idea, the fixation will slowly become less and in time will transfer to the person of the therapist, the ecclesiastical authority, and ultimately back to the parents. This process then renders the God-idea free from pathological ideation and open to healthy development.

As an example, in the case of a patient with severe religious conflict, the transference remained fixated on the God-idea, while the transference problems in relation to the mother were transferred to the female therapist and members of the group. During this period, the patient made steady improvement. There was, however, insufficient relief of his feelings of guilt and rebellion in his religious life, which was in direct relationship to some seriously delinquent behavior. After two and a half years, he was transferred to a male analyst for individual therapy hours.

From the first session, his relationship with the male analyst showed all the rebellion and hostility he had had in relation to his God-idea. It was difficult to persuade the male therapist to keep him in treatment because of the severity of the negative transference, but because he remained in group therapy with the female therapist, she was able to encourage him to continue. At the time when the patient came in to treatment with the female therapist, he had no apparent relationship with his father, although the childhood history indicated that there had been a relationship with him in childhood. As a result of the female therapist's efforts, the patient developed a warm and happy relationship with his father in the present and worked through his hostility towards his mother. After several months of his hostile transference to the male therapist, he also began to be hostile and rebellious with his father. Thus, the religious conflicts, which were severe in the experience of the female therapist, were so jarred free of the God-idea and transferred onto the male therapist and back to the father that the male therapist did not see the patient as a problem of religious conflict.

A closely allied phenomenon of parent transference onto the God-idea is seen in cases of strong reaction formation in which the God-idea is all good and the parent is all bad—or vice versa. These people will deny any part of the hated transference, but in the course of the analysis of behavior problems or psychosomatic illness it becomes apparent that the God-idea is just too good or just too bad, and slowly it becomes apparent that the patient has two God-ideas, one in consciousness and the opposite in repression, but operative. In one case, the real father was at times good, loving, and devout; at other times, he was an angry, cruel, guilt-ridden backslider in a very severe fundamentalist denomination. In another case, there were two fathers—the bad biological father and the very good father-substitute the patient found in his pastor.

Both these examples stand primarily as evidence that the therapist must attack the religious problem head on, using the religious representation as a starting point for psychoanalytic exploration. However, this does not imply that all religious problems can best be solved exclusively in analysis of basic human problems and conflict. When the therapist can find his patient a good confessor, he will be astonished at the amazing working through of guilt that can occur in this sacramental action. The analyst who has spent months of hard work preparing his patient to accept the emotionally valid sacramental absolution will be deeply gratified and rewarded. In those denominations that do not use confession, other religious rituals may be equally effective. Yom Kippur can be such a confession experience for the Jew whose therapist has taught him to make use of it.

The author has seen a patient, in his fifties, who had a remarkable turning point in the relief of a dangerously severe depression when a courageous and devout priest made use of his sacramental authority and baptized this patient. It was a symbolic realization that someone wanted him and loved him. Both the therapist and the religionist are often prone to undervalue these sacramental acts. A devoutly sincere blessing, touching the head with the hands, can comfort a troubled or dying patient.

At the present time, our most effective clergy in these areas are frequently our well-trained chaplains, especially chaplain supervisors. However, the presence of such persons should not reinforce the shyness of the therapist to work as "spiritual director." Such a role in a therapist sensitive to and educated in work with the religious person, in my opinion, is no more inappropriate than sexual counseling seemed some years back.

Psychotherapists who are inexperienced in work with the religious person can fail to make use of one of the most recognized therapeutic tools: direct release of feelings toward an object that may not necessarily be the one that originally elicited the feelings. An excellent example lies in depression, when many patients feel and express serious distortion of religion; analysis and use of antidepressant drugs are appropriate but not necessarily sufficient. The patients feel an estrangement from God. They are angry with Him and become mute in their rage (will not pray). The therapist may encourage direct expression of the anger to God, which for most Christians is forbidden and hence very difficult. When achieved, however, improvement occurs. Such direct expression to God is easier with Jews, who have a tradition of talking to God about their anger with Him, as well as expressing their grief, sorrow, and weeping in prayer [1, 2]. The fundamentalist can be shown Leviticus 19:17, "Thou shalt surely rebuke thy neighbor and not bear sin because of him," and St. Paul, Eph. 4:26, "Let not the sun go down on your wrath," as meaning not repression or suppression, but working it through. Also, Jesus was often angry, as when he cleared out the Temple. With these people, words such as *annoy-ance and righteous indignation* are more acceptable than anger and hostility [1, 3].

A Lutheran has great difficulty in his anger with God theologi-cally; this can be by-passed by explaining that he is only angry with the transferences that distort his awareness of the "otherness" of God.

In summary, we may say that the success of psychotherapy with religious personnel is primarily a function of the therapist's acumen in understanding those idiosyncrasies of religious conviction that are carriers of pathologic ideation. Such understanding lays the groundwork for creative analytic responses that touch on the pa-tient's unconscious message without having to obliterate the con-scious manifestations in religious thought.

It can be helpful to follow the psychoanalytic psychic entities in culling out religious conflict. Prominent among examples would be the distortion of the God-idea with fierce superego demand and punishment [2]. Some patients reason that their very need for psy-chotherapy stands as evidence of God's unforgiveness [1]. They im-ply that prayer alone should elicit God's forgiveness, meaning that their sins are of a greater order than can be healed by prayer. A childlike God-idea is a ready-made carrier of the merciless discon-tent of the superego. Patients who have a good and mature religion ("I am not alone or abandoned, He is with me") have a better prognosis than those with a belief in an angry, cruel, punishing, and whimsical God, who heals or hurts as His fancy dictates. The prognosis is poor until and unless such a malevolent God-idea can be changed to a good, mature, and growth-inducing one in the course of therapy.

Ego function can also be relegated to the God-idea. Here we see the patient who maintains early dependent fixations in his current personal relationship with his God. Psychotherapy, the strengthen-ing of the coping ego function, of existential responsibility, as it were, can only succeed as the patient is freed of magical expecta-tions of his God's intervention in outer reality. He must come to accept the apparent unpredictability of most of natural law.

Although the treatment of religious personnel is admittedly diffi-cult and requires some special techniques and freedom from coun-tertransference to religious ideation, in some respects the religious population is easier to treat than the layman. The professional religious tend to have greater emotional investment, and therefore conscious concern, in their religious conflicts. Since these conflicts carry so much deeper material, the patients are, in this sense, well motivated. As a group, these people are set apart. With the arma-mentarium of special interest on the therapist's part, the free and creative use of individual and particularly group therapy [4], I can say from the experience of treating many that significant gains can be made.

The importance of creative but controlled intervention cannot be overemphasized. A Roman Catholic layman never accepted the Episcopal clergymen in his group as really priests, but this was not apparent until a Roman priest came into the group as an invited guest, and then the religious conflicts of this layman exploded in hours of verbal hostility towards the Roman Church and the ig-norant, bigoted parish priest of his childhood and his teachings, which could only be corrected by the authority of this mature Roman priest in the group situation.

The author works under the premise that any religious person who needs therapy has religious conflicts. The presenting symptoms may be psychosomatic, behavior problems, or thinking disorders, either neurotic or psychotic. Magical thinking is quite common, even in solidly neurotic religious personnel. Concretization of thinking, with loss of ability to understand abstract thinking, espe-cially as in poetry, is often quite difficult to treat in religious per-sonnel and is a very serious problem in all religious conflicts. Sexual problems range from heterosexual inhibition to promiscuity, homo-sexuality, impotency, and so forth, as in all laymen.

When not handled with the deep acceptance of the reality of religious ideation, the psychotherapy experience can be one more constricting and isolating experience for these already lonely per-sons. When handled in the spirit in which I have tried to present the material of this paper, it can lay the groundwork for both the relief of deep pathology and the liberation of creative, healthy religious experience [7, 8].

REFERENCES

1. Bowers, M. K.   Protestantism in its Therapeutic Implications. *Annals of Psychotherapy Monograph No. 2.* New York: American Academy of Psychotherapists, 1959.
2. Bowers, M. K.   *Conflicts of the Clergy.* New York: T. Nelson, 1963.
3. Bowers, M. K.   Passive submission to the will of God. *Past. Psychol.* 16:11, 1965.
4. Bowers, M. K., Berkovitz, B., and Brecher, S.   Therapeutic implications of analytic group psychotherapy of religious personnel. *Int. J. Group Psychother.* 8:243, 1958.
5. Bowers, M. K., Jackson, E. N., Knight, J. L., and Le Shan, L. *Counselling the Dying.* New York: T. Nelson, 1964.
6. Fulton, R. E. (Ed.).   *Death and Identity.* New York: Wiley, 1965.
7. Otto, R.   *The Idea of the Holy.* New York: Oxford University Press, 1923.
8. Psychiatry and religion: some steps toward mutual understanding and usefulness. *Group Advance. Psychiat. [Rep.]* 48, 1960.
9. The psychic function of religion in mental illness and health. *Group Advance. Psychiat. [Rep.]* 67, 1968.

PART IV
CLINICAL COLLABORATION
OF CLERGY AND MENTAL
HEALTH PROFESSIONALS

This section takes up the innovative and experimental work that is being carried out by clergymen and psychiatrists. This work is a reflection of both the developments in clinical pastoral training and the developments in community psychiatry. Thus here, theoretical questions aside, the clergyman and the psychiatrist come together in their mutual concern for the treatment and nurture of the mentally ill.

Pattison outlines some of the opportunities for case-finding and case-referral by the clergy, yet notes some of the current obstacles. He goes on to suggest new roles for the clergy in community mental health centers, as well as in mental health primary prevention in the community. Knights reports on role changes occurring in chaplaincy work in mental hospitals. He suggests means for maximizing the functions of the chaplain as a professional team member. Draper discusses the very human problems met with in providing useful psychiatric consultation to clergymen. He points out some of the pitfalls for both psychiatrist and clergyman and some of the values that accrue from such consultation. Boverman describes his own experiences in collaborating with a clergyman in psychotherapy, and expands his discussion to general principles that the psychiatrist can use in working with the clergy in direct clinical treatment. Then Midelfort describes a variety of settings in which the psychiatrist can work with church organizations, church officials, and individual clergymen in meeting a variety of mental health needs.

These chapters point up some of the problems in status, communication, and role differences that lie in the way of effective clinical collaboration. They also provide examples of how successful collaboration has been and can be carried out.

The Role of Clergymen in Community Mental Health Programs

E . M A N S E L L P A T T I S O N

INTRODUCTION

The importance of clergymen and churches for mental health programs was brought to national attention by the studies of the Congressional Joint Commission on Mental Health and Illness during 1956 to 1961. These reports indicated that clergy were a primary and major mental health resource. As a consequence, strong recommendations were made for intensive collaboration between mental health professionals and the religious community. This collaboration was held to be especially crucial for the development of community mental health centers [9, 15, 18, 24].

This chapter will review the major findings that formed the basis for these recommendations, survey the degree to which such program implementation has occurred, and discuss some implications for the future. The chapter will be divided into three areas of distinctive function for the clergy: (1) the clergyman as a primary case-finding and referral agent; (2) the clergyman as a primary-care agent and primary prevention agent; (3) the clinically trained clergyman as a professional team member in a community mental health center (here abbreviated CMHC).

THE CLERGY AS CASE-FINDING
AND REFERRAL AGENTS

The Joint Commission survey of national mental health resources revealed that when people felt emotionally distressed they
preponderantly turned first to a clergyman: 42% saw a clergyman,
29% a doctor, and 18% a mental health professional [9, 18]. There
are a multiplicity of reasons why clergy are chosen. Clergy are the
most numerous of professionals (350,000 in the U.S.), they are
widely scattered so that they are geographically accessible, they are
easy to contact at any time, they are less expensive, their role and
function are usually well known so that people know what to expect, and they have ongoing contacts already established with many
people, so that in times of crisis it is natural to turn to them.

The survey also revealed that people in distress were looking for
someone who could give them comfort, advice, support, and reassurance. Most people were not seeking changes in themselves, but
rather were looking for emotional support. The data suggest that
people see the clergy as helpful, making few demands on the person in distress, whereas mental health professionals are more apt
to give less immediate assistance and demand more on the part of
the distressed person. The survey also revealed that clergymen are
successful in terms of client satisfaction: 65% of clergy-clients were
satisfied compared with 45% of psychiatrist-clients. Again, 18% of
clergy-clients were dissatisfied compared to 24% of psychiatrist-
clients.

There are many variables behind these bare statistics, yet they
still remain an impressive demonstration that clergymen are among
the most important care-taking agents in the community. They are
in a position to play a vital role in *secondary prevention,* i.e., early
case-finding and effective early referral for treatment.

How well do the clergy currently fill the role of secondary prevention? It is estimated that over one-third of clergy-clients suffer
severe mental illness. Yet the clergy refer only 33% of such severe
cases to psychiatrists, whereas general practitioners refer 88% of
such cases [23]. In terms of total case contacts, several recent sur-
veys demonstrate that clergy refer *less than 1%* of their contacts to

mental health resources. Alternatively, data from mental health services reveal that only 1 to 8% of their referrals come from the clergy [4, 13, 17, 18, 19, 23]. Even in newly established community mental health centers the figures are minimal. In the recent monograph on eleven model community mental health centers, I found the following level of clergy referrals: St. Vincent's, 2%; Einstein, 1%; Prairie View, 4%; Nebraska, "few" [20, 21].

Such findings have stimulated recent research studies to determine why the clergy have not become an effective part of the secondary prevention network of referral [3, 19, 23]. First, there is a marked discrepancy between role definitions and role functions of the clergy as defined by psychiatrists and as defined by the clergy. Psychiatrists tend to restrict and confine the role of the clergyman and even voice grave warnings about clergy assuming professional functions or encroaching on psychiatric domains. Conversely, clergymen define their role and function with broader scope, authority, and competence. When clergymen do accept the restrictive psychiatric definition, they tend to avoid referrals which would "show them up" or "expose their inferior status."

Second, psychiatrists do not usually treat clergymen as part of a professional colleague relationship. Piedmont [23] recently demonstrated that psychiatrists rarely acknowledge referrals from clergymen and rarely transmit usable information about a patient back to the referring clergyman, even when requested to do so. Elsewhere, I have documented examples of CMHC that have established clinical intake policies of accepting only medical referrals and deliberately excluding clergy referrals [20]. This has certain screening advantages and may help integrate the medical community, but it is also a powerful deterrent to the clergy.

Third, clergy referral tends to vary with the security, training, and social status of the clergy. Clergy from low-status peripheral denominations refer very few people because of their social distance from psychiatrists, whereas high-status clergy refer at a much higher rate. Fourth, referrals vary with clergy definitions of health and illness, and the degree of disparity perceived with psychiatry. Clergy with the least formal training and the most conservative theology tend to define all emotional problems as spiritual and attempt to deal with the problem in the least psychological manner. When these clergy refer patients, it will usually occur because mental health professionals are personally known who are sympathetic to religion. Conversely, the most educated clergy, usually of liberal theology, have tended to have high rates of referral. They define most emotional problems as psychological and may even eschew any sort of spiritual approach [10]. Interestingly, a "new breed" of ministers is now appearing, ministers who have had extensive clinical training. These clergymen have redefined their role as capable caretakers who have knowledge, skill, and responsibility for the direct care of their people. These clergy have lower referral rates because they feel that they are just as capable of dealing with many problems as mental health professionals [2].

In sum, the clergy are on the front line of our communities in serving the mentally ill. They are in an ideal position to implement secondary prevention measures in terms of early case-finding and effective referral into the triage system of mental health treatment services. To date our community mental health programs have *not* capitalized on the clergy as resource for a variety of complex reasons. More effective use of the clergy requires the following: (1) extensive education of the clergy, both in seminary and in service, in the field of mental health and in how to work with mental health professionals; (2) extensive education of mental health professionals in the structure, function, and role of clergymen and church institutions and in how to collaborate with clergymen; (3) the development in both professional groups of clearer role definitions and role boundaries, with guidelines for establishing effective referral networks; and (4) reevaluation of community mental health programs so that effective referral relationships can be established between CMHC and the clergy in the community the CMHC serves.

THE CLERGY AS PRIMARY-CARE AGENTS AND PRIMARY PREVENTION AGENTS

As noted above, the clergy see a preponderance of those who are emotionally disturbed in the community. Ten years ago, emphasis was placed on helping the clergy to be more effective referral agents. However, that was at best only a partial answer. If the clergy did refer all their contacts to mental health professionals, with already overcrowded offices and clinics, we would be jammed and swamped!

More recently, community mental health programs have sought to distribute the responsibility for mental health care more widely over the community. Thus, programs have been developed for education and consultation to primary-contact agents. The intent is to increase the skill, sophistication, and willingness of primary-contact agents to assume *continued-care responsibility* for the emotionally distressed in the community. The goal of such *indirect* mental health programs is to *decrease* overall referrals and *increase* *selectivity* of referrals from primary-contact agents to specific mental health service systems. This means that clergy should be taught and assisted in the task of caring more effectively for the large number of people seeking pastoral help [15, 24].

This movement in community mental health programming dovetails with educational and vocational changes occurring in the clergy. Since World War II, the field of pastoral psychology has proliferated rapidly, producing two distinct professionals: (1) the trained chaplain, and (2) the pastoral counselor. The chaplain, as a specialized role, is not of direct concern here, as our focus is on the clergyman in the church.

Much of the early pastoral counseling movement was devoted to a fairly wholesale aggrandizement of psychological theory and psychotherapeutic techniques. The movement flowered into the American Association of Pastoral Counselors, whose membership requirements bore strong resemblance to that of a psychoanalytic institute. As might be expected, this generated strong controversy both within pastoral education and with mental health professionals [19]. An attenuation of this direction appears to have occurred as pastoral counselors have sought to redefine their role as a specialized ministry of the church, rather than just assuming counseling skills. Further, such advanced clinical training seems most applicable only in large churches, which can afford such a special staff, or in urban settings, where multiple church support is available [12, 14].

A third direction has developed in the past five years, namely, an emphasis on training the pastor in the pulpit. The emphasis here is not on the acquisition of complex clinical skills, but on an enrichment of pastoral skills so that the pastor can have basic counseling knowledge and skills as part of his armamentarium. The pastor in this instance does not assume a counselor role, but rather he counsels and helps his parishioners with increased expertise within the role, traditions, and functions of the church pastor. Instead of pastoral counseling, we now speak of this as *pastoral care* [2].

This brings up an important clinical issue that has received little study to date. Heretofore, we have often assumed that primary-care agents were merely secondary substitutes in lieu of sufficient mental health professionals. But the issue now is *when and with whom* may the primary-contact agent, such as the pastor, be the *preferred therapeutic agent*. In fact, work is now going on to define the unique characteristics of pastoral care, its advantages and disadvantages, as a distinct mode of therapeutic help.

A second major role of the parish pastor lies in the area of *primary prevention* in mental health, namely, the promotion of positive mental health. This is an area yet largely unexplored in terms of a scientifically verified base for action, yet it is of great theoretical import to the development of social and community psychiatry. The church is a major social force in society. Through its teachings, activities, and relationships, human potential can be either inhibited or maximized [1].

The pastor can play a determinative role in the emphasis and impact of a church institution on its members, as well as on the larger community. First, through his preaching, the pastor may foster either a neurotic, destructive view of self or a healthy, mature view of self and others. As one minister remarked after a consultation seminar, "I can see that I've been tearing my people apart on Sunday morning and trying to patch them back together during the rest of the week." Second, the church can provide primary groups that offer intimacy, support, and relationship. Many churches have been developing small group programs as a major mode of participation in the church. Some such groups approach therapeutic goals, whereas other such groups are aimed at affording a primary reference and relationship group so necessary for maintaining interpersonal well-being. Other group programs are geared to the needs of specific groups, such as young people, old people, middle-aged single adults, divorcees, or servicemen. Such groups often not only serve the members of the church, but also reach out to and involve many other persons in the community. Third, the church can provide material and human assistance to people during life crises —the age-old tradition of helping people in distress. With increasing urbanization and population mobility, increasing numbers of persons have few contacts to whom they can realistically turn when in crisis. Both the pastor and his church may provide a revitalization of this traditional function recast in terms of the mental health emphasis on effective crisis intervention. Fourth, the clergyman and his church can be an influential resource in the community in response to social problems of concern to the whole community. This intersects with the concerns for social action that community mental health programs face in many communities where mental health programs interdigitate with health, education, and welfare problems.

To maximize the above functions of the clergy, the following needs appear: (1) the development of theoretical and clinical skills in pastoral care, addressed to the pastor in the pulpit; (2) training and consultation programs to clergy to assist them in implementing church programs that will maximize mental health values; and (3) active collaboration between community mental health programs and churches in their communities when faced with social issues of joint concern requiring mutual action.

THE CLERGY AS PROFESSIONAL
TEAM MEMBERS IN CMHC

With the development of the mental health chaplain, a new dimension of pastoral function was added. Boisen established the first training program for mental health chaplains back in the

1930's, and gradually the role of the chaplain in various institutional settings has been established. Various studies have demonstrated that currently there is a continuum of chaplaincy roles, ranging from providing religious programs, to being an ancillary staff member, to being an integral team member of a total institutional program [8, 16]. To date, however, little attention has been given to the specialized roles that a clinically trained clergyman might play in the newly developing CMHC [22].

For example, in the monograph on model CMHC, none of the eleven CMHC list a chaplain or clergyman as a staff member, although in three CMHC there was a pastoral consultant for exclusive work with ministers [21]. The two church-related CMHC make no mention of chaplain activities! Doubtless there are chaplaincy activities at all eleven programs, but we may assume that the role is peripheral and ancillary to the CMHC programs. It would seem that if the clergy and the church are to be cultivated as a major mental health resource, more attention will have to be given to the role of clergy in CMHC programs. I will outline four functions that a clinically trained clergyman may well play in a current CMHC.

Function 1:   Director of Pastoral Care

This function involves the usual religious activities that ministers provide: religious services, administering the sacraments, individual pastoral calls, and so forth. Traditionally, each faith group has been concerned about the ministry to the spiritual needs of its adherents. Hence, chaplains at times have been held suspect by their pulpit colleagues for deserting the specific ministry of the church and working in a secular setting, where proselytizing and specific dogmas are inappropriate [11]. The chaplain has a responsibility to the entire patient population and the therapeutic program as a whole. As such, he can implement religious programs that do not have specific theological aims but are therapeutic in intent. We might call this "generic religious work." Since religion is fairly ubiquitous and religious activities often serve important social and communicative needs, we might view such religious work as therapeutic, although not therapy. Recent theological discussion has sought to develop a theological base for such generalized religious service of the chaplain. Such pastoral care is thus seen as part of the redemptive healing concern of the church to all people in distress. In addition to directing such generic religious activities, the chaplain may well serve specific spiritual roles and, in addition, coordinate and supervise the work of visiting clergy, who might volunteer to work with their parishioners who are patients in the CMHC.

Function 2: Consultant in Psychotherapy

Here, the chaplain would still function in his pastoral role, but would shift his focus to that of assisting in specific treatment processes. The chaplain here may counsel with a patient concerning theological or spiritual questions, offer support during periods of stress or anxiety, help the patient fit his religious background into his therapeutic experience, and participate in religious rituals that may therapeutically benefit the patient [6, 8]. As more attention is given to religious values in psychotherapy, the chaplain may also serve as a consultant and interpreter to the psychotherapist in regard to religious concerns of the patient. As more religious persons seek psychotherapy, it may be that the relevance of their religious background will require more attention in diagnostic and therapeutic evaluation.

Function 3: Diagnostic Consultant

Here, the chaplain would function as an expert on religious matters. The chaplain thus becomes a member of the diagnostic therapeutic team [7]. The chaplain may interview the patient and explore the patient's religious life as part of the diagnostic evaluation [5, 25]. As an expert on various religious cultures and with knowledge of the role of religion in personality, the chaplain is in a position to offer relevant insights for a psychodynamic diagnosis and for appropriate use of religious resources in the community for rehabilitative purposes.

Function 4:   Liaison to the Religious Community

Here, the chaplain moves into a role that capitalizes upon his clerical identity, religious knowledge, and contact and identification with the religious community. The chaplain may carry on education and consultation programs for clergy and churches in the community. Likewise, he may conduct teaching seminars on religious aspects of mental health for the staff of the CMHC. In his liaison role, the chaplain would be a primary agent in developing and maintaining liaison between the CMHC and the churches. This would include developing a referral network and assisting in arranging after-care and rehabilitation programs for patients, in which clergy and churches could participate. The need here is for a clergyman-chaplain who is thoroughly familiar with the treatment of the mentally ill. He must be able to communicate easily and meaningfully with psychiatrists, psychologists, social workers, and others on the mental health team, as well as with the clergy. He must, in effect, have thorough training in the mental health field. Such training should enhance his professional skills as a minister, but his role should not be exclusively that of a pastoral counselor. He should be an expert in both mental health and religion, and should be the specialist in the field who brings these special skills to the full-time staff of the CMHC as a fellow professional.

In sum, there are a variety of interlocking roles that a clinically trained clergyman can play in the CMHC. The employment of such clergy in CMHC with full professional status affords an avenue for fuller implementation of the religious resources in the community in CMHC programming [20].

SUMMARY

This chapter has outlined the front-line role that clergy play in the mental health picture of the community. A great deal of work needs to be done with both clergy and mental health professionals if the clergy are to be appropriately used in the role of referral agents. Attention will also have to be given to CMHC referral policies. The clergy are in the process of developing skills in the area of primary-contact care. Education and consultation programs provided by mental health professionals are needed in this area, as well as in promoting the primary prevention function of the clergy and the church. Finally, there is need for the development of specialized chaplain roles and functions in the CMHC if the religious resources of the community are to become an integral part of comprehensive CMHC programming.

REFERENCES

1. Clinebell, H. J., Jr. *Mental Health Through Christian Community.* New York: Abingdon, 1965.
2. Clinebell, H. J., Jr. *Basic Types of Pastoral Counseling.* New York: Abingdon, 1966.
3. Cobb, A. R., Main, R. L., and Pierce, C. M. Barriers in pastoral counseling research. *Ment. Hyg.* 49:337, 1965.
4. Cumming, E., and Harrington, C. Clergyman as counselor. *Amer. J. Sociol.* 69:234, 1963.
5. Draper, E., Meyer, G. G., Parzen, Z., and Samuelson, G. On the diagnostic value of religious ideation. *Arch. Gen. Psychiat.* (Chicago) 13:202, 1965.
6. Fritze, H. P. Pastoral counseling with a patient in psychotherapy. *Bull. Menninger Clin.* 16:136, 1952.
7. Gluckman, R. M. The chaplain as a member of the diagnostic clinical team. *Ment. Hyg.* 37:278, 1953.
8. Gross, G. A., and Fritze, H. P. The function of a chaplain in psychotherapy. *Bull. Menninger Clin.* 16:136, 1952.
9. Gurin, G., Veroff, J., and Field, S. *Americans View Their Mental Health.* New York: Basic Books, 1960.
10. Haas, H. I. Relations between clergymen and psychiatrists. *Psychiat. Quart.* [*Suppl.*] 1:1, 1967.
11. Hadden, J. K. A study of the protestant ministry in America. *J. Sci. Stud. Relig.* 5:10, 1965.
12. Johnson, B. The development of pastoral counseling programs in Protestantism: A sociological perspective. *Sociol. Rev.* 1:59, 1958.
13. Kennedy R. J., and Linsky, A. S. Attitudes and Activities of

the Clergy in the Area of Mental Health. Unpublished manuscript, University of Washington, 1965.

14. Klausner, S. Z. *Psychiatry and Religion: A Sociological Study
of the New Alliance of Ministers and Psychiatrists.* New York:
Free Press, 1964.

15. Knight, J. A., and Davis, W. E. *Manual for the Comprehensive Community Mental Health Clinic.* Springfield, Ill.:
C. C. Thomas, 1964.

16. Knights, W., and Kramer, D. Chaplaincy role-functions as seen
by mental patients and staff. *J. Past. Care* 18:154, 1964.

17. Larson, R. F. Clerical and psychiatric conceptions of the
clergyman's role in the therapeutic setting. *Soc. Prob.* 11:419,
1964.

18. Larson, R. F. Attitudes and opinions of clergymen about
mental illness and causes of mental illness. *Ment. Hyg.* 49:52,
1965.

19. Larson, R. F. The clergyman's role in the therapeutic process:
Disagreement between clergymen and psychiatrists. *Psychiatry*
31:250, 1968.

20. Pattison, E. M. Functions of the clergy in community mental
health centers. *Past. Psychol.* 16:21, 1965.

21. Pattison, E. M. Review: The community mental health center.
Past. Psychol. 16:55, 1965.

22. Pattison, E. M. Clergymen's role in community health clinics.
J.A.M.A. 203:182, 1968.

23. Piedmont, E. B. Referrals and reciprocity, psychiatrists, general practitioners, and clergymen. *J. Health Soc. Behav.* 9:29,
1968.

24. Westberg, G. E., and Draper, E. *Community Psychiatry and
the Clergyman.* Springfield, Ill.: C. C. Thomas, 1966.

25. Wiedeman, G. H. The importance of religion: Sectarianism in
psychiatric case study. *Amer. J. Psychother.* 3:392, 1949.

The Role of the Chaplain in Mental Hospitals

WARD A. KNIGHTS, JR.

INTRODUCTION

The last several decades have ushered in a new era of concern, on the part of organized religion, for those persons who are patients in our mental hospitals. This concern is primarily expressed in the provision of appropriately trained clergymen who have come to work as chaplains. This new expression of religion's interest in the institutionalized person is now well established in relation to mental hospitals as well as in regard to other types of institutions. It has been in existence long enough that there has been opportunity for research and study of the role of the chaplain [2].

RESEARCH CONCERNING THE CHAPLAIN'S ROLE

Two reports of research help to set forth the role of the chaplain as it is perceived in clinical situations.

In 1960, Gynther and Kempson [6] reported the results of their work in assessing objectively the attitudes of patients and staff toward the developing chaplaincy program at the South Carolina State Hospital. It was shown that staff in general thought of chaplains as counselors, while patients viewed them as preachers. Education, administration, and evangelism were not seen as being important. There were considerable differences within the hospital staff in regard to how the chaplain's activities were perceived. Nurses were least favorable to the activities of the chaplain, aides held the most favorable attitudes, and the medical auxiliary and physicians obtained intermediate scores. In general, it was concluded from this study that even though there was general approval of the work of the chaplains, the real motives and goals of the chaplaincy program were often misunderstood. There were conflicting expectations of chaplains' functions that stood in the way of more adequate functioning.

Gynther and Kempson also reported a tendency for staff members who were themselves religious to look favorably on the chaplain's work. Those who did not consider themselves religious were less favorable. Religious involvement on the part of staff members seemed to vary with status. The higher his status, the less interest the staff member showed in religion. This raises a question not answered in this study: To what extent do staff members project their own religious needs, or lack of them, onto their patients, thereby ceasing to be truly professional in their own functioning in relation to the religious needs of the patient?

In 1964 the role of the chaplain was studied at the Cleveland (Ohio) Psychiatric Institute [10]. Fifteen actual or possible role functions were investigated, which gives an indication of the variety of role functions of the chaplain in the mental hospital. These fifteen were (1) leading religious worship, (2) administering sacraments, (3) making general visitations, (4) counseling with patients, (5) visiting the physically ill, (6) teaching in in-service programs, (7) relating to the community, (8) conducting clergy training, (9) performing administrative functions, (10) teaching formal religious classes, (11) participating in research, (12) performing disciplinary functions, (13) working with volunteers, (14) counseling with employees, and (15) doing religious group work.

Of these role functions only one, performing disciplinary functions, did not represent a current function of chaplains in mental hospitals and was not included in job descriptions. This list was not considered to be exhaustive in terms of actual duties performed.

The results of this study showed that leading religious worship and visiting patients were functions of the chaplain perceived positively by more than 90% of both the staff and the patients. The only other function that received such a highly favorable response was that of administering sacraments, which was rated quite positively by the staff but much less positively by the patients. All of these functions are, of course, highly traditional ones for clergymen, yet they represent only a fifth of the total number of functions that were investigated. Much less favorable ratings were given to the nontraditional functions. Compared with other staff members, the medical staff (psychiatrists and physicians) consistently showed the least favorable perception of the less traditional functions. This was true also in regard to the traditional functions.

Another interesting finding of this study was that the patients seemed to look more favorably than the staff on the teaching role of the chaplain. Again this causes us to question the accuracy with which staff members assess the needs of patients in terms of pastoral care.

In general, this study indicated that while there was a good acceptance of the chaplain in the mental hospital, acceptance was in regard to very limited traditional role-functions. The nontraditional functions, which actually made up the bulk of the chaplain's work, were not understood and were, at best, only nominally accepted.

It is not possible, of course, to say to what extent the two studies cited reflect accurately the situation of the chaplain in mental hospitals across the country. It is assumed, however, that the results reflect typical situations.

NONTRADITIONAL ROLE FUNCTIONS

The nontraditional role functions of chaplains can be grouped in three primary categories: (1) teaching and research, (2) administration, and (3) therapy.

Teaching of other professionals and research are nontraditional in the sense that they have not been typical functions of the parish clergyman. It must be noted, however, that in contemporary society the functions of the clergy have undergone drastic changes. The traditional pastor is now more a myth than a reality. The activities of the clergy have become diversified and specialized. Current thinking in regard to theological education is tending toward a dual role of pastor and theological educator for many clergymen who serve a local congregation [15]. Such a role is illustrative of the kind of radical departure from the stereotype that has taken place and is still continuing today. Some forms of research, as that term is understood by the psychological sciences, have become basic to the very structure of many religious bodies, and increasing numbers of clergymen are trained in research methods as part of their graduate education. The chaplain not only is part of this general broadening within the field of religion but represents a specialization in terms of his particular interest. Many chaplains, having had extensive academic and clinical training, become teachers of other clergy and ancillary professionals. The function they serve in this role is part of the reason for their presence in the mental hospital.

The participation of the chaplain in research is often considered an appropriate and important activity. Such involvement seems especially appropriate for the chaplain in the mental hospital, since this setting offers him a unique opportunity to study the "living human documents" in a way that is not available to the parish clergyman.

Administrative duties may be mentioned as a nontraditional activity of chaplains, because although all clergymen serve to some degree as administrators, this aspect of their functioning is usually overlooked. The planning of training programs and the relationship with clergy, church groups, and social groups outside the hospital often consume more of the working hours of the chaplain than is realized. When the chaplain's participation on various committees and in other hospital functions is also considered, it can be seen that administration constitutes a very large part of his work.

The therapeutic functions of the chaplain represent, perhaps, the greatest departure from the traditional role. Yet here, also, as in the teaching and research functions, the chaplain reflects the new stance of organized religion, which has appropriated for itself the insights in relation to human behavior that have come from the psychological and social sciences. This acceptance has been not merely academic, but also functional. It is not at all unusual for clergymen to be graduates of psychoanalytic institutes, and today a great many clergymen receive some form of clinical pastoral education as part of their theological education.

Nearly all chaplains today have had specialized training in addition to their usual theological education, and most have had parish experience before coming into chaplaincy work. Therefore, it is the rule rather than the exception for the chaplain in the mental hospital to be trained as a counselor using modern psychotherapeutic procedures. Many chaplains may also have been trained to do group psychotherapy. In general, it may be said that most chaplains are conversant with, and capable of using, modern psychotherapeutic techniques in their relationships with mental patients.

Another function of chaplains that may perhaps best be considered nontraditional is the pastoral function of the chaplain in relation to the institution. While this role has not been traditional for chaplains, it must be said that it has been for clergymen in their parishes. The parish clergyman, be he priest, rabbi, or minister, has always found a primary role in a general "shepherding" of the organization he has served. He has provided general leadership and guidance for all type of activities, from baked bean suppers to the involvement of his parish in the civil rights movement. He has had general concern for all his people in all their involvements in life from birth to death. This same broad concern for people and their involvements is carried over by the chaplain into the mental hospital as part of his professional identification. He is therefore prepared for broad participation in relation to the concerns of the mental hospital.

CLINICAL COLLABORATION

As a number of writers have recently pointed out, there currently exists little understanding at the grass roots level between clergymen and psychiatrists [3, 7, 12]. This is probably less true of chaplains in mental hospitals than of clergymen in general. Yet even here, aspirations run far ahead of actual collaboration, in spite of all good intentions to the contrary. Draper [3] makes the interesting observation that competent members of both professions are always found to be collaborating. If this is true, then it is surely a much-needed comment on the lack of maturity in both professions.

Actual clinical collaboration can exist only when professional prejudices are set aside and professional functioning is viewed in a dispassionate manner. For an example of the extent to which unreasonable professional identification has been allowed, in the past, to generate irresponsible attitudes, we may note one psychiatrist who, in a textbook on psychotherapy, says: "Indeed, *all* physicians, *whether they know it or not*, practice psychotherapy . . ." [14] (emphasis added). A little later in the same book he says: "With rare exception however, ministers are *not* equipped to enter into any kind of therapeutic program . . ." (emphasis added).

While the chaplain in the mental hospital might be considered one of the "rare exceptions," the prejudicial nature of these statements tends to impede collaboration rather than promote it. If left unchecked, this eventuates the attitude that says: "Only a medical background prepares the professional for an understanding of the human mind . . ." [14]. Such an attitude is unacceptable, of course, to any clergyman and would be, also, to most other professionals. The blanket inclusion of *all* of one professional group in the circle of the elect and the blanket exclusion of all but a *rare exception* from certain other groups smacks of the kind of paternalism that is a betrayal of the inadequacies in the system that generates such attitudes. A similar attitude has also existed, of course, within the ranks of clergymen. However, this attitude has been rare among chaplains.

At this point, we shall assume the maturity of both professions and suggest that there are three main areas in which there may be clinical collaboration between psychiatrist and chaplain in the mental hospital. For simplicity, we shall label these areas as those in which the chaplain functions (1) as a diagnostic consultant, (2) as a consultant in psychotherapy, and (3) as a religious therapist.

The Chaplain as a Diagnostic Consultant

Because of his knowledge of religion and through his experience and training, the chaplain is in a position to gather and interpret information in relation to the patient's religious life that can be of great value to the psychiatrist as he seeks to arrive at a diagnosis. With the increasing emphasis being placed on values and their interpretation in psychotherapy, such diagnostic consultation will increase in importance.

There have been a number of interesting and informative reports in regard to actual situations in which chaplains have been members of diagnostic teams, one of which is the report of Stein and Thomas [13]. The importance of consultation in relation to the patient's religion becomes especially important when the psychiatrist is of a different religious faith than his patient. In such a situation, it would be impractical for the psychiatrist to visit the patient's church to ascertain its religious life, or to study the sacred books of the religion to gain an understanding of its teachings, or to study its history and theology. As desirable as such activity might be for broadening the psychiatrist's understanding of a particular religion, it is quite impractical when the psychiatrist is faced with his diagnostic responsibility. As an expert on religious matters, the chaplain stands ready to offer information on religious teachings and practices and also to offer a special kind of insight into the relationship between religion and personality [4].

If such clinical collaboration is to become a reality, there will have to be more attention given, in the training of the psychiatrist, to religion and its place in personality. With such training, the psychiatrist will see the need for consultation and will have a frame of reference that will allow him to utilize the information once it is obtained. Changes will also have to come about in administrative procedures. One type of change that will be required will be in the official forms that are utilized in patient records. While in the majority of hospitals there are appropriate forms used by all departments within the hospital, there are usually none for the use of the chaplain. Therefore, both chaplain and psychiatrist labor under an administrative handicap that puts a large block in the way of their collaboration.

Closer collaboration in regard to diagnosis will mean not only personal consultation between chaplain and psychiatrist, but also closer relationships with the entire "healing team." Where diagnosis is determined primarily through staff conferences, the chaplain will have to be accepted as a functioning team member by the psychiatrist in charge of the team. As Golden [5] has shown through his research, chaplains tend to fulfill those functions that administrators expect them to fulfill. If there is to be collaboration in regard to diagnosis, there will need to be considerable initiative shown by those psychiatrists who function as administrators, as well as by the staff psychiatrists.

The Chaplain as a Consultant in Psychotherapy

As a patient's psychotherapy is planned and carried out, close collaboration between psychiatrist and chaplain may be advisable in many cases. Besides his contribution to the diagnostic process, the chaplain is in a position to give continuing advice in regard to religious concerns. This may be done in consultation with the psychiatrist, or the psychiatrist may deem it more desirable for the chaplain to work directly with the patient in the religious area, according to carefully predetermined plans mutually arrived at by psychiatrist and chaplain.

In many instances, there is a need for a strong supportive relationship for the patient between individual sessions with the psychiatrist. The chaplain, in fulfillment of his basic pastoral role, is in a position to offer very strong support because of his identification with religion. The chaplain, as all clergymen, finds a basic identification in empathic relationships with persons, as Johnson [9] has so clearly pointed out. This identification may be appropriately used by the psychiatrist to give support to patients at appropriate points in their therapy.

There will also be need, in the therapeutic process, for the patient to reintegrate his religious experience into his experience as a patient. It is at this point that the chaplain can also function appropriately as consultant.

The chaplain may serve not only as a consultant to the therapeutic process, but also as a supplement to such therapy. In one situation, for example, chaplains helped to translate insight into action for many patients when they took them to churches to help reestablish social and religious contacts in the community. Those patients who had gained insight into their social isolation through individual and group psychotherapy were thus given the complementary experience through which they could begin to utilize their insight to take appropriate action [11].

It may be added, of course, that the traditional religious ministries, themselves, may appropriately be utilized to implement psychiatric goals. One particular aspect of treatment, the aspect that focuses upon guilt, becomes a particularly appropriate focus for collaboration. Here, the traditional practices or sacraments that deal with guilt may be utilized for the enhancing of the treatment process of the individual patient, under the psychiatrist's direction.

The Chaplain as a Religious Therapist

Up to this point we have considered the chaplain as primarily in collaboration with the psychiatrist. Now we shall consider the chaplain in a role that will require the psychiatrist to perform the services of a consultant. We shall consider the chaplain as a religious therapist, or as he is perhaps more appropriately called by the religious community, a pastoral counselor.

In order for the psychiatrist to be willing to function as consultant to the chaplain in this role, he must be willing to admit the limitations of his own position as a representative of the modern mental health movement. His position in this movement greatly restricts the relevance of his relationship to the total life of any person. As Howland [8] has pointed out, the modern mental health movement is based on a conception of mental health that subordinates religious concerns.

Such a subordination can never be accepted by religion. Religious people can never accept the subordination of their religious life to what may perhaps best be called *secular* concerns.

It is the personal conviction of this author that the main reason for the lack of collaboration between psychiatrists and chaplains is the outrageous presumption on the part of the mental health movement that has subsumed and subordinated religion. Only as this presumption is changed will there be any real rapprochement.

The chaplain functioning as religious therapist has his own unique goals for his relationship with the patient. As a clergyman, he enhances his primary goal with modern techniques and insights that help him establish a truly therapeutic relationship with the patient.

It should be noted here, also, that the chaplain's therapeutic relationship with patients is by no means limited to those who express overt religious concern. As Boyer [1] found in his research, the value of the relationship the chaplain offered to the patient depended more on the quality of relationship that was offered in the immediate confrontation than on the previous "religiosity" of the patient.

As the chaplain pursues his work as religious therapist, he will quite appropriately seek consultation with the psychiatrist in those areas in which the psychiatrist possesses unique insights. The pattern for such collaboration has been set in pastoral counseling centers, which have been increasing quite rapidly in the past decade. In these centers, the pastoral counselors function as therapists with the advice of psychiatrists and other professionals.

Since the model is available, it would seem a tragedy if such active collaboration should not become more widespread. Particularly in mental hospitals, where the human need is so great, and where the staff is chronically insufficient to give the kind of care that should be given, the active collaboration of psychiatrist and chaplain serves only to bring greater benefit to the patient.

REFERENCES

1. Boyer, R. R.   An Exploration into the Nature and Use of the Concept of the Healing Team in Fairview Park Hospital. Un-

published manuscript, Oberlin Graduate School of Theology, 1962.
2. Carrigan, R. L.   The hospital chaplain, research, and pastoral care. *Past. Psychol.* 17:39, 1966.
3. Draper, E.   *Psychiatry and Pastoral Care.* Englewood Cliffs, N.J.: Prentice-Hall, 1965.
4. Gluckman, R. M.   The chaplain as a member of the diagnostic clinical team. *Ment. Hyg.* 37:278, 1953.
5. Golden, E. S.   What influences the role of the Protestant chaplain in an institutional setting? *J. Past. Care* 16:218, 1962.
6. Gynther, M. D., and Kempson, J.   Attitudes of mental patients and staff toward a chaplaincy program. *J. Past. Care* 14:211, 1960.
7. Holt, H., and Winick, C.   Psychiatry, religion and self. *Past. Psychol.* 19:35, 1968.
8. Howland, E. S.   The unique contribution of the clergyman to health. *J. Past. Care* 21:91, 1967.
9. Johnson, P. E.   *The Psychology of Pastoral Care.* New York: Abingdon-Cokesbury, 1953.
10. Knights, W. A., and Kramer, D.   Chaplaincy role functions as seen by mental patients and staff. *J. Past. Care* 18:154, 1964.
11. Knights, W. A., and Langheim, I.   Re-introducing religion. *Staff* 3:6, 1966.
12. Pattison, E. M.   Functions of the clergy in community mental health centers. *Past. Psychol.* 16:154, 1965.
13. Stein, L. I., and Thomas, J. R.   The chaplain as a member of the psychiatric team. *Hosp. Community Psychiat.* 18:197, 1967.
14. Wolberg, L. R.   *The Technique of Psychotherapy.* New York: Grune & Stratton, 1954.
15. Zimmerman, J. S.   The relevance of clinical pastoral training to field education. *J. Past. Care* 22:1, 1968.

Psychiatric Consultation to Clergymen

Not much more than 25 years ago, psychiatric consultation to the helping professions, including to medical specialties other than psychiatry, was a stereotyped affair, often geared only to diagnostic or dispositional goals. Lawyers asked, "Is this man crazy?" "Can he distinguish right from wrong?" "Can he stand trial?" Other physicians of hospital staffs queried, "Can he be transferred to a psychiatric ward?" "Is he committable?" "Is he suicidal?" "How should he be sedated, hypnotized, or controlled?" On the other hand, the tradition of the clergy has been to ask, "What are a man's motivations?" "What is the nature of man?" "What makes him tick?" "What is in his heart?" [11] With the maturation of dynamic psychiatry, the clergy's quest for answers in understanding man's behavior found, at first, a reluctant source in psychodynamic psychiatrists.

The pastoral care movement, pioneered by many, including Anton Boisen [1], himself a victim of schizophrenia, began its pursuit like a "hound of heaven" of dynamic psychiatrists. Clergymen in quest of understanding and guidance for pastoral work, and eventually for training, supervision, and instruction, gradually became specialists of the ministry within the general pastoral care movement of the church. A revitalized investment in pastoral work with the individual brought the clergyman to the dynamic psychiatrist's door with the request, "Can you help me understand and provide for my parishioner?"

For a few uncertain years, the dynamic psychiatrist, flushed with his popularity as a modern wizard, feared entrusting to a medical layman, professional though that layman was in another sphere, the potent knowledge of psychological understanding. Although Freud clearly indicated his hope that psychoanalysis be utilized by pastoral workers, and shared much with the Reverend Oskar Pfister [14], eager young theologians in the 1940's and 1950's were looked upon suspiciously as intruders in the field of mental health. That is, they were until the onset of psychiatry's "Latter Day Social Gospel" [15, 16] in the form of community psychiatry. Clergymen suddenly became care-takers of prime importance for community psychiatrists' purposes. The pendulum had swung, and the seekers became the sought! [2]

To complicate the picture still further, the church was experiencing its own reassessment. After a quarter of a century of great interest in understanding and helping the individual, it, too, has turned to social issues with new vigor. Its young blood finds excitement and challenge in community organization, racial issues, revision of social structure, concern for the masses, and group processes. In the meantime, psychiatric consultation has become myriadic, ready to offer undreamed-of varieties of services.

This admittedly oversimplified evaluation does offer some context for fingering the texture of the clerical cloth that psychiatric consultation attempts to weave itself into, is woven in, or is patched on. However, so that oversimplification does not lull us to sleep, a few modes of interaction and varieties of consultation might be mentioned.

I would admit to having had a rather unusual degree of investment in the area of psychiatric consultation to clergymen, hardly typical of most psychiatrists. Having passed from pre-med to a transient interest in medical missions, to ministerial training with its renaissance in pastoral counseling, to medicine, to psychiatry, and finally to psychoanalysis, my training life carried through the pendulum swings mentioned above. I had the privilege of being tutored by and then sharing professional interests with a number of luminaries in the field of pastoral care, including Carroll Wise, Richard Dicks, Granger Westberg, Seward Hiltner, and last but not least, the distinguished theologian, Paul Tillich. My consultation-ships have been to Christian and Jewish theological schools; to pastors' workshops as far away as Fairbanks (with Carroll Wise) and as interdisciplinary as those of the Academy of Religion and Mental Health and the Cornell Research Planning Workshop of 1961 [3]; to research and training operations, e.g., the Kokomo-LaGrange projects with Granger Westberg [17]; to pastoral coun-seling centers such as those of Chicago's Metropolitan Church Federation; to mission boards (Baptist and Methodist); to various chaplaincy programs; to study groups, e.g., the one sponsored by the World Council of Churches; to multiple staff ministries; to groups of ministers seeking special training; and to individual ministers in a supervisory capacity. I mention these not so much credentially as inferentially; i.e., there are nearly infinite varieties possible for consultation to the church and clergy. I know per-sonally of psychiatrists and psychologists who act as consultants for dioceses, bishops, church administration, religious education direc-tors and programs, pastoral counseling organizations, church plan-ners, and on and on. There are well-established organizations with special interests in psychiatric consultation, such as the Society for the Scientific Study of Religion, the Academy of Religion and Mental Health, the American Association of Pastoral Counselors, the committees on religion of the American Psychiatric Association, the American Medical Association, and the Group for the Advance-ment of Psychiatry.

What mention of all these is leading up to is this: the futility of particularizing psychiatric consultation to clergymen. My own work has ranged well into prosaic consultative roles (working with mental health centers, institutions for the physically and mentally handicapped, child and family agencies, general physicians, chil-dren's institutions, mental health zone centers, universities, etc.). But, there are, I believe, principles that can be outlined under three categories of attitudinal problems that present some hazard to consultants. Freud [8] pointed toward three instinctual wishes that are "born afresh with every child. . . . Among these instinctual wishes are those of incest, cannibalism and lust for killing." Acted out, these wishes form a triad of the great crimes that man is capable of perpetrating against his brother. Sublimated, these present special problems in consultation.

Cannibalism. What I mean by cannibalism is the inclination to ingest, consume, or subsume another's theory of man's nature and behavior (a clergyman's theology) into one's own personal philosophy without so much as "by your leave." As I believe we have clearly shown in an earlier study [7], a man's personal philosophy (his private view of man and life) is just that, personal and individualized. His own life experiences have molded his *weltanschauung.* In this sense no one is "orthodox." Yet each of us is sensitive to another's subtle attempt simply to incorporate our personal views into his gastric system. Our intellectual self, which has natural narcissistic investment, resists "silent preachers" who exhort us under the guise of "translation" or "clarification" [10]. Whereas we psychiatrists seem to have emancipated ourselves at least to some degree from the temptation to subsume an artist and his productions into our personal theory [12], we have not yet shown such freedom in the realm of philosophy and religion. In this arena, we are more inclined to say (or if not "interpret," feel) "Oh, I know what you mean. All you are really talking about is the Oedipus complex." With that, the distinctive and separate elements of that person's religion are well on their way past the hard palate. Although religionists may have this problem, too, it is an acknowledged and conscious part of their role to bring others to their point of view. For them, too, however, this need not be a process of digestion. (For a counterpart to psychiatry's cannibalistic tendencies toward religion, see McClelland's article [13], which labels psychoanalysis a religion in disguise.)

More specifically, the consultant's early task is to establish a contract that is consciously mutually satisfactory and as quickly as possible learn the "unwritten contract" in order to handle its ramifications. For example, a minister may appropriately seek supervision, but his latent goal is treatment or referral. A church body may ask for didactic courses but unwittingly seek a powerful outside authority to deal with an administrative conflict. A skillful consultant will not thus be content to "explain dynamics" but will use his knowledge both to meet the conscious expectations of his employer and to use his interpersonal assets and psychological skills to maintain his role as consultant. If he views religion as disease alone, without integrity, validity, and autonomy, he becomes attitudinally a therapist or evangelist, not a consultant. As a consultant, his own philosophy requires security sufficient to allow another *his,* using techniques of illumination, not obliteration. It is one thing to share an insight that enlarges the perspective of a consultee. It is another to require him to hang the new perspective on the consultant's personal life format.

A related cannibalistic tendency of the neophyte consultant is to insist on cramming his "goodies" down the throat of his consultee. Although one might consider this imposition close to rape or fellatio, its assumption is still related to the cannibalistic conviction that *the* system of thinking that *really* holds water is the consultant's. This leads to didactic excursions that "teach" canned psychodynamics, psychiatric diagnosis, and jargon. The diagnostically astute consultant might have discovered that his clergyman's more pressing problem than a need for psychiatric information, for instance, was his reluctance to assess his parishioner as objectively as possible, lest he be "judgmental."

Appreciation of the special problems of pastoral counselors as contrasted to those of other professionals doing psychotherapy will include different kinds of function and identity peculiar to pastors. The clergyman's model of the structure of interpersonal work will vary tremendously. The pastor rarely, if ever, terminates with a parishioner. For those of his flock who mean the most to him, this applies even in spite of a geographical move. The clergyman's life has fishbowl characteristics. His anonymity is locally absent and his professional role puts a tax on finding good friends with whom he can share deeply with freedom. (Ministers' wives have perhaps even larger hurdles in this regard [4]). Besides his community visibility, he will perform multiple functions that bring him into intimate, revealing, formal, or business contact with his counselee. For an analyst the "rule of abstinence" (which fundamentally requires him to have in good check his narcissistic returns from patients) is a "hard saying" to clergymen.

Incest. In contrast to cannibalism, consultative incest is the urge to mate at all costs, "just so we stick together." The consultant's unresolved philosophy or religious identification may prompt him to find, too quickly, "brothers under the skin." He may search out and find pastors as allies whose goals are "humanitarian" (too often a catchword for a vague union). "After all, we are all working for the same common cause. Really now, aren't the differences between our points of view pedantic?" This inclination is not always the clergy's problem. For instance, following a paper at a large and distinguished psychiatric hospital, I heard a discussant begin his remarks with, "We all know that psychoanalysis is a Jewish science."(!)

The problem here rests largely with those consultants who cannot feel free to differ, those whose philosophical views are fuzzy, or those who have not yet worked through a brainwash. A consultant's objectivity and realistic self-appraisal ought to insure for him the ability to assert a "not me" position, the courage to acknowledge real differences, and the ability to distinguish the psychiatric body of scientific knowledge from mergers that get sanctified into pseudo religions. Part of a Rogerian holdover that fits passivity traits in certain ministers is a readiness to listen, to placate, to win friends and influence people at the cost of professional identification. Chaplains, in particular, have subjected themselves to the "permissive" role of being everybody's friend—often at the high cost of prostituting themselves.

One can see the *defense* against incest or "mixing blood" in the "untouchables" of clergy and psychiatrists. "Never the twain shall meet" has counterparts in both professions. Dr. Maxwell Gitelson's unfortunate presidential message of 1962 [9] compares "favorably" with certain religionists' insistence on a unilateral orthodoxy. Both positions smack of unresolved and defended concerns over psychological incest. Realistic sharing of perspectives and amalgams without deification that prove fruitful become preempted.

Murder. Although cannibalism implies the death and consumption of a similar species, it may not necessarily imply murder by the cannibal himself. Fortunately, consultant contracts usually are not made if a murder contract is likely. Mutual exploration is common practice and definitely worthwhile to screen impossible matches.

Murderous wishes may develop if either party enters the arena of unbridled competitive ambition. As physicians, we have known facets of the medical model that may not have useful application in consultation. One is the inclination or willingness to take over. Another is the discomfort associated with the problem of leadership when ancillary colleagues are not only useful, but perhaps pivotal. As a consultant to clergymen, it is the psychiatrist who is ancillary. A psychiatrist friend of mine, whom I respect highly, had begun to recognize that entirely too much of his time was spent in consultantships. These did not really further his own ambitions nor, as far as he could tell, did they make significant program alterations in the agencies that hired him. His creative talents, capable of molding a significant child psychiatry program, were being diluted, dissipated, and frustrated as he spread himself thin. "As a consultant, I became 'His Majesty, the Baby.' I believe I have a contribution to make and it will require my full attention and responsibility." He realized, as some consultants do not, his strong wish to run the show, his own show. It was time to stop consulting. He is now running his own show, and well. Had he remained the consultant with persistent wishes to "do it better" than his administrative employer, the consultee, there might have been psychological murder or its alternative, isolation. Few consultants successfully run someone else's show. If they do, someone is inadequate or psychologically impotent.

Although I understand my friend's point about "His Majesty, the Baby," my own experience has been closer to "His Majesty, the

Prince," and not crown prince or heir apparent. In none of my consultations to religious bodies or social agencies have I posed a serious threat to the power of actual leadership. Yet extraordinarily rewarding results of consultation made this exciting activity worth the effort; consultative gratification came not only in the forms of teacher's pleasure, income, diversity of professional activity, and "red-carpet" treatment, but in program alterations that did reflect mutual investment in shared goals that left role integrity intact.

Community psychiatry consultants are learning a hard lesson. Community alterations of significance come from the leadership within, not through superimposed artificial plans or dreams of outsiders, including psychiatrists. Although dynamic pastors with leadership capacities have earlier sought psychiatric consultants, many are now edgy. The eagerness and even evangelism of community psychiatrists who blatantly call clergy "care-takers" along with hosts of other community leaders arouse apprehension in the local parish. If the psychiatrist then does not come to learn and identify with community needs, but only to organize, preach, or teach, his consultative power is doomed. No sincere clergyman has as his primary goal becoming an agent of mental health.

Perhaps the earliest recorded account of consultation is to be found in Genesis (chapters 41 to 50). After a number of harrowing experiences, including false accusations that landed him in jail, Joseph had developed a reputation as a dream interpreter. Pharaoh, having his problems, found out about the young Hebrew's accuracy and gave Joseph a consultative audience. After nailing down a 14-year prediction of first feast, followed by famine, he counseled Pharaoh about program. Joseph's apparent humility, accuracy, and willingness to give God the credit put him "up front." Joseph had told Pharaoh he needed a "discrete and wise man" to set over Egypt. It just so happened that such a man was Joseph! Pharaoh's ring, possessions, treasures, stewardship of rule, a high priest's daughter, and the Pharaoh's *second* chariot all became Joseph's. Even his father, Jacob, and his brothers took his counsel and prospered through Joseph's talents. Very carefully, however, Pharaoh made it clear from the beginning that "only in the throne will I be greater than thou" (Genesis 41:40). Not too subtly he reminded Joseph, "I am the pharaoh." Things prospered for Joseph, his family, and the children of Israel in Egypt until Joseph's death, when a new administration took over. "The new king knew not Joseph" (Exodus 1:8), and that meant trouble. Although Joseph broke a few consultative rules, like becoming the indispensable man, Pharaoh and he did keep power issues straight, with mutual benefits and long tenure.

A basic commodity we offer the church and clergy is an understanding of mental functioning, human behavior, motivation, emotional conflicts, and principles of healing. This professional knowledge and our experience should enrich the clergy's appreciation of religion's meaning and potential. Its function as a human resource [5], its potency for attracting psychological cathexes [6], providing tranquilization, control, social change, inspiration, and creativity make consultation a productive, rewarding art.

REFERENCES

1. Boisen, A. T. *Out of the Depths*. New York: Harper, 1960.
2. Caplan, G. *An Approach to Community Mental Health*. New York: Grune & Stratton, 1961.
3. Cook, S. W. (Ed.). *Research Plans in the Fields of Religion, Values and Morality*. New York: Religious Education Association, 1962.
4. Douglas, W. *Ministers' Wives*. New York: Harper & Row, 1965.
5. Draper, E. Religion as a Human Resource. In *Psychiatry and Pastoral Care*. Englewood Cliffs, N.J.: Prentice-Hall, 1965.
6. Draper, E. Psychological Dynamics of Religion. In this volume.
7. Draper, E., Meyer, G., Parzen, Z., and Samuelson, G. The diagnostic value of religious ideation. *Arch. Gen. Psychiat.* (Chicago) 13:202, 1965.
8. Freud, S. The Future of an Illusion (1927). In *The Complete Psychological Works of Sigmund Freud* (Std. ed.). London: Hogarth Press, 1961, Vol. XXI.

9. Gitelson, M. Communication from the president about the neo-analytic movement. *Int. J. Psychoanal.* 43:373, 1962.
10. Hartmann, H. *Ego Psychology and the Problem of Adaptation.* New York: International Universities Press, 1958.
11. Kierkegaard, S. *Purity of Heart Is to Will One Thing: Spiritual Preparation for the Office of Confession.* New York: Harper, 1956.
12. Kohut, H. Beyond the bounds of the basic rule. *J. Amer. Psychoanal. Ass.* 8:567, 1960.
13. McClelland, D. C. The New Church of the Unconscious. In *Princeton Bulletin,* 1958.
14. Meng, H., and Freud, E. L. (Eds.). *Psychoanalysis and Faith: The Letters of Sigmund Freud and Oskar Pfister.* London: Hogarth Press, 1963.
15. Rauschenbusch, W. *Christianity and the Social Gospel.* New York: Macmillan, 1912.
16. Rauschenbusch, W. *A Theology for the Social Gospel.* New York: Macmillan, 1917.
17. Westberg, G., and Draper, E. *Community Psychiatry and the Clergyman.* Springfield, Ill.: C. C. Thomas, 1966.

Psychiatrist-Clergy Collaboration in Psychotherapy

MAXWELL BOVERMAN

INTRODUCTION

For some time I have been particularly interested in attempting constructive psychotherapy with the psychotic patient so as to avoid calamitous hospitalization. Some of the technical problems involved led to my initially working with the clergy. The case presentation in this chapter has been reported in an earlier paper [1], as an example of professional collaboration used to deal with common problems in the treatment of a psychotic patient.

My experiences have led to the development of an expanded social view of the patient. Working at first in the context of individual, psychoanalytically oriented psychotherapy, modifying therapeutic techniques thought suitable for neurotic patients by use of increased therapist activity, confrontation, reality testing, support, and so forth, I found it possible not only to engage some extremely ill patients in therapy outside the hospital, but also to achieve some favorable results in altering disturbed patterns of living. However, these were mainly highly motivated patients who came to treatment voluntarily. They had, regardless of their severe symptomatology, an optimum basic ego strength and a capability for forming a good therapeutic relationship. As the criteria for acceptance for therapy became less strict, I realized that there were certain limita-

279

tions inherent in the design of the individual treatment situation. No matter how refined the theoretical understanding of the patient's psyche or how the therapeutic technique was altered, certain patients who had initiated therapy and had seemingly established a workable therapeutic relationship would break off treatment inexplicably. This often appeared paradoxical, because they seemed to be improving. In addition, many patients, although remaining in therapy, simply did not improve as expected. A good deal of information showed that a major factor in determining the course of therapy was the influence of certain "significant others" in the patient's life—family, teacher, friend, pastor, etc. They were thought of as "sabotaging" treatment, a notion of some validity but naive and oversimplified in its concept of blame and limited in its applicability because of the planned isolation of the therapeutic relationship. Naturally, the "nonpatient" psychotic person had to be considered as untreatable until, unfortunately, he was so disturbed as to justify his removal from the community to a hospital.

Starting in the 1950's, studies of families with a sick member by the Don Jackson group, Lyman Wynne and his colleagues, Murray Bowen, Nathan Ackerman, and others, demonstrated the pathological illness-producing life styles, interactions, and communications characteristic of the whole family. By the same token, studies of groups and various social milieus, such as those by Schwartz and Stanton and Maxwell Jones, demonstrated psychosis as consequence of, or influenced by, a particular social system. Along with these investigations came techniques of therapy, e.g., family therapy, based on constructive intervention in a system, thus enlarging the possibilities of treatment being applicable to any significant person(s) within the system and not being limited to the identified patient.

Around this time, I was being referred patients for treatment by the Pastoral Institute, an agency to which pastors turned for assistance with parishoners' emotional problems. In addition, a consultative role brought me even more in contact with the problem of the nonpatient, the person or family with a significant psychiatric disability whom it was impossible to refer for realistically available therapy. I became acquainted with this problem as seen within the religious institution of the parish and thus became interested in the existence and characteristics of the patient-family-pastor-parish social network and in how this network might encourage illness or be useful in promoting health in the event of illness. I became increasingly impressed with the fact that the church not only was important ideologically in the lives of many people, but was a social community of special significance, as yet relatively unappreciated in its psychiatric possibilities.

It was against this particular background, in which we had just begun to think about the social context of emotional illness, that I first met the Reverend James R. Adams, a young, perceptive Episcopal priest who was attempting to cope with a serious parish and family crisis involving a psychotic woman and who was willing to invest some curiosity and personal risk. This situation, in 1961, led to our working together in what was probably for me, and undoubtedly for him, the first intentional acknowledged and direct pastor-psychiatrist collaboration in psychotherapy. Although we did not realize it at the time, this effort offered a paradigm for a kind of collaborative effort in psychotherapy.

CASE REPORT

In the fall of 1961, a professional staff member of the Pastoral Institute called me to see if I would accept for treatment an acutely psychotic woman who had been seen with her husband for evaluation. This 40-year-old housewife had been gradually withdrawing and acting a little "odd" for several years. Within the past several months she had periods of complete withdrawal alternating with episodes of bizarre emotional storms within the family and publicly, showing religiosity and evidence of hallucinations and persecutory delusions. Both husband and wife had involved an increasing number of people who were in contact with their helplessness, confidences, troublemaking, and openly psychotic behavior. In addition, they made direct demands for help of different kinds from their pastor, fellow parishoners, neighbors, family physician, another physician, relatives, a psychiatrist, a psychoanalyst, and another minister. Previous professional recommendations for treatment had been ignored, and the patient refused to return for therapy after consultation with a psychiatrist prior to my being called.

I believed that any consultation with this woman or her husband would be fruitless because of their already apparent irresponsibility, involvement of others in their problems, and previous refusal of competent professional assistance. One possible approach would be to intervene in the social network that appeared to be supporting or at least tolerating this chaotic state of affairs, so as to confine the illness and enhance motivation for change. Other than the sick couple, the only interested and responsible person available to me was the referring pastor, Mr. Adams, and I called him prior to any consultation with the patient. He and I discussed the poor prognosis of this situation based on the history of difficulties in attempting therapy, and I frankly told him that I was interested in the problem only if I could be assured of his being involved closely in an experiment with some possible risk and discomfort. The tone of our discussion then, as later, was informal, frank, pragmatic, concrete, and as specific and realistic as possible.

When the husband called for the first consultation, he stated that, while he would attend, *he* had no problem—his wife was the sick one and needed help. I saw the couple together and, after obtaining the history, discussed my opinions: The problem was a serious one; there was a need for psychiatric treatment; there were both indications for and disadvantages of hospitalization and serious risks involved in maintaining such a severely ill patient outside a hospital. Contributing dynamics were hostile denial and ambiguity, and an important part of the process was the husband's passivity and irresponsibility. The family either could hospitalize the patient, or, if they wished to pursue treatment outside an institution with me, could do so on a private basis in a program that would include family sessions.

In requesting help, the couple presented a destructive stalemate by setting down some impossible conditions. The husband had planned to start a new and more responsible job in a distant city within a few weeks, leaving his sick wife in charge of the family while the children completed their education; he would return on weekends. He refused to revise his plans to deal with the family crisis. He insisted on putting his wife under my care without participating in the treatment program, and asked for reduced and delayed fees, claiming impoverishment. I felt that not only was the husband avoiding assuming responsibility, he was possibly afraid that the new job was beyond him, and he and his wife were in collusion to rescue him from this job or the responsibility of possible failure by using her illness as a handicap, which it would have been.

A series of telephone conferences was held with the pastor, resulting in his later intervention in several anticipated disruptive crises commonly seen in psychotherapy. We agreed that we would be in frequent touch with each other, especially if there were developments of which the other might not be aware. The patients were informed of our relationship. The pastor was helped to recognize subtle hostility, avoidance of responsibility, manipulativeness, and other destructive behavior in the family and its social network. He was encouraged to notice and confront those involved in this appalling situation, but only when he felt it possible as a pastor and friend. Both husband and wife were to be faced with their joint responsibility for their misbehavior and the chaotic situation, and the pastor was encouraged to be aware of his feelings and appropriately to express displeasure directly and unambiguously.

I encouraged openness between the pastor and the family's friends, suggesting that the pastor could invite conversation about this situation, thus obtaining information about the family's behavior. Friends should be encouraged to be forthright and to confront rather than indulge or be falsely sympathetic when confronted with hostile exploitation. I hoped to break up a cycle of pseudomutuality by making the family uncomfortable when they were acting destructively. Hopefully, this confrontation would avoid the usual consequences of polite indulgence or tolerance of misbehavior with subsequent avoidance and isolation of the family.

Following the initial consultation, the wife refused to return for treatment, and the husband attempted to engage me in accepting his conditions, at first by telephone and later in my office. He returned to his pastor, and I discussed with his pastor his irresponsibility and manipulativeness in this as well as some other situations the pastor had reported to me. As a result, Mr. Adams and some involved parishioners changed their approach; instead of being dishonestly sympathetic and comforting or distantly polite, they expressed dissatisfaction directly with the couple, and were pleased and grateful with the new experience of confronting the family and the family's response.

Within a week, the husband arranged for the treatment program as recommended, consisting of biweekly sessions involving the entire family, including a 17-year-old son and a 15-year-old daughter. Individual psychotherapy was suggested but proved unproductive and was not pressed. Family therapy consisted of pointing out the pathological behavior as seen in the schizophrenic family with various other techniques of intervention.

Early in treatment, the husband said that his wife was now well, as an attempt to justify stopping therapy. The pastor had direct information that contradicted the husband's statement, and this information was utilized in confronting the family and avoiding a familiar treatment crisis. The husband then attempted to discontinue therapy because of finances. I insisted that the wife (who still appeared quite psychotic at times and opposed treatment) get a job to help, but only after I talked with the pastor and received his support. When her husband not only agreed but insisted, and we threatened to exclude her from the family meeting, she got a job and has been working satisfactorily since.

Several weeks later, the pastor informed me that the wife had been discussing her delusions with neighbors and also was spreading derogatory stories about me. This was interpreted as a hostile manipulation to gain sympathetic allies and to embarrass the family. This behavior discontinued after it was discussed with the family and they responded with disapproval, and the wife seemed to be doing quite well.

The husband then threatened to hospitalize his wife, saying that she was getting sicker. I had ample concrete information from the pastor to indicate that, in fact, she was working and getting along quite well socially, so I was able to explore the matter further. Actually, the husband was piqued because she had been acting coldly toward him, and hospitalization was not considered further.

In the fourth month of treatment, the patient attempted suicide while her husband was out of town. She used drugs obtained from her physician, who had been asked both by the husband and by me not to treat her psychiatric problem with drugs. On taking the drugs, the patient called her neighbor, who then called Mr. Adams. He did not go to the house but instead called me. The problem of suicide had been anticipated and discussed frankly in the family sessions, and a plan of action had been laid down in terms of this being a family responsibility, with the son being appointed head of the family if father was away and mother incapacitated. The pastor called the son, who came home immediately from his nearby school and arranged for immediate hospital treatment for the drug poisoning, and the patient returned home that evening. The father was called and was enraged, as were the children, and he insisted she return to work the following day. The neighbors, encouraged by the pastor, expressed not only their concern but also their annoyance and disapproval. In response, she openly displayed the rage that had been dormant and possibly had led to this attempt. This was another crisis that could have led to hospitalization but that was averted by the pastor's assistance.

Following this incident, the behavior of the family seemed more open and direct, and there were no more crises, although a number of problems remained unresolved. Treatment was discontinued after six months at the husband's request. I continued to receive reports from the pastor about the family's state. The wife was doing quite well, with no psychotic behavior; the husband's social behavior, some of which had been quite objectionable, had improved, and he seemed more responsible; but both children still seemed somewhat spoiled. Obtaining such early follow-up information would ordinarily be unique and could only have been done easily by the pastor.

In 1963, a year after the first consultation, the wife, for the first time, called me for an appointment for herself. She had been depressed following the son's joining the Army and had cut her wrists in a suicidal gesture. We met several times individually, and the couple were then seen for almost a year in a psychotherapy group of married couples. During this time, their relationship was tempestuous, but she showed no signs of psychosis and continued her work, and the couple showed some improvement. When her husband received a promotion offer, she again made a suicidal threat, and for a time the husband seemed more interested in investigating his problems.

Both Mr. Adams and the couple left the original parish; he to go to another church, and they to change from a house to an apartment because the children had now left the family. A brief telephone follow-up with them in 1967 revealed that there had been no further suicidal attempts, overt psychosis, hospitalization, or incapacitation, both parties working satisfactorily. They felt that the treatment had been very helpful and continued to be useful to them. The wife has, for some time, seen another psychiatrist, only occasionally. The couple still express some dissatisfaction with their relationship, but are apparently settled in it; their daughter lives alone and is working and pursuing an artistic interest; the son has married and has two children, and is regarded as somewhat dominated by his wife.

DISCUSSION: PRINCIPLES OF COLLABORATION

Clergymen and psychiatrists may collaborate in psychotherapy in different ways. Supervised by the psychiatrist, the clergyman may be the primary therapist and treat the patient himself; he may be an assistant or additional therapist, treating the patient alternately with the psychiatrist (sometimes done for economic purposes); or he may be a secondary therapist, such as a social worker, treating another member of a family, with the psychiatrist treating the primary patient. These models, while they may be useful, are not especially different from the usual mental health professional treatment team. The attempt at collaborative effort described in this situation is the working together of psychiatrist and pastor *complementarily*, with both parties acting in accordance with their specific role functions, using the techniques, resources, and capabilities appropriate to the different professions, and recognizing the limitations of each.

One of the principles of this collaborative effort is the process of *clarification of roles* in terms of acceptable, rational, appropriate behavior and assumption of responsibilities and opportunities. For example, in the given case, the family's responsibilities were defined, and the assumption of these responsibilities by others was discouraged. The pastor did not, as is commonly done, undertake psychotherapy of the sick person refusing therapy, nor did the fellow parishioners undertake being nursemaids or scapegoats. The psychiatrist was able to provide therapy when retained, and was also involved in a consultative role to the pastor and parish. The pastor, both in his ordinary pastoral duties and in his counseling interviews, was able to be helpful. He did not, however, assume the professional behavior of the psychotherapist or the role functions (e.g., medical responsibilities) of the psychiatrist. Therefore, his participation was *complementary* rather than as an additional psychiatric professional.

The study of *communication* necessarily accompanies role clarification. Various destructive types of communication, especially hostile vagueness and ambiguity, which result in isolation and rejection of the psychotic member, were seen and attempts were made to change them. The process not only includes the pastor in relation to the patient, but also utilizes his resources in being in contact with other members of the parish network. We attempted to interrupt destructive ambiguity, hostile denial, and the secondary gains of illness by making open and explicit that which was implied, pressuring and enabling the people to make conscious choices and discouraging rewarding of sickness.

An important part of the collaboration is the pastor-psychiatrist relationship. It is necessary that communication between the two be simple, unambiguous, educational, and thereby effective. Criticisms about psychiatrists not offering anything useful are not always evidence of resistance and may be quite true.

The relationship was openly acknowledged, and there was an explicit statement that we would not hold to the usual confidentiality of individual treatment; both Mr. Adams and I were free to discuss at our discretion anything we knew about the family. This is a question that concerns the professional workers, but apparently not the patients. Actually, confidentiality considerations are usually honored in the breach in many situations of this kind, and to observe them would have made for an impossible task. Those matters that were discussed openly had very little to do anyway with the giving of confidential information, but rather concerned public interactions between various people.

One important aspect of the collaborative relationship was its ongoing nature. In this case, the relationship lasted throughout the period in which the case was the responsibility of either of us. But the relationship is also ongoing in that this case has led to the development of further collaborative efforts to the present. Rather than being an isolated professional incident, this should be viewed as part of an educational and developmental process in which both parties participated, utilizing their previous experiences, expertise, and resources. Both of us felt free to use what we had learned in the past, and also to call upon each other when a new problem arose in the present. I believe the educational aspects are mutual. The cleric has information about the patient, his family, their social lives and religious ideology, and the leverages and limitations of the church institution. The psychiatrist contributes technical data about diagnosis of illness and kinds of destructive behavior. In addition, he assists the pastor as a person by assisting his development both intellectually and in the recognition and effective handling of his feelings.

INDICATIONS FOR COLLABORATION

The indications for (and quality of) the pastor-psychiatrist collaboration depend in part on the nature and intensity of the pastor-family relationship. There is a difference between a patient referred by a clergyman he has never or only formally met, and a family with whom the pastor has, so to speak, lived.

It is well to recognize that when a person is referred by a pastor (especially if the parish is not large), they well may be neighbors and mutually participate in the parish social and worship activities. They probably have been involved in the crises of ordinary life as well as the neurotic ones, and the pastor has probably held some counseling sessions with the family. This indicates a uniquely significant relationship of some intimacy and investment, containing qualities of family, neighbor, professional caretaker, religious advisor, and spiritual healer, as well as friend. The potentials for a continuing involvement of the pastor in the sickness, with possibilities of hostile competitiveness, feelings of rejection, manipulativeness, and so on, are not only great, but are not likely to be interrupted by a doctor's order to stop seeing each other.

Conventionally, the problem of hostile passive dependency is dealt with in psychotherapy by the device of an exclusive relationship that resists the distracting maneuver of engaging others in the relationship. Including others in the treatment, therefore, is something not to be undertaken lightly and without a realization of possible disadvantages, such as relieving the patient of his responsibility for his cure. Unfortunately, the simple fact remains that many people with significant psychiatric handicaps simply will not even initiate therapy themselves, let alone carry it through successfully.

The criteria that are commonly thought of as necessary for psychotherapy are high motivation, intelligence, ability to tolerate anxiety and resist acting-out, a reasonable ego, ability to form a therapeutic relationship, a life situation that does not completely prevent change, and the lack of secondary gains or rewarding of illness in the environment. Therefore, when the patient does not possess the criteria for establishing a separate, responsible, and successful therapeutic relationship, it is justifiable and necessary that the referring pastor be brought into the picture.

Factors indicating a lack of suitability for reliance solely on the individual patient and calling for the pastor's participation are, for example, previous crises that involved the pastor and others; a pattern of irresponsibility; serious illness, e.g., psychosis ordinarily difficult to treat; poor motivation for therapy; previous patterns of acting-out, especially with imposition on others; the pastor's continuing involvement in the problem, seductively or otherwise competing with the psychiatrist; continuing manipulativeness by either the patient or the pastor; exhaustion of the pastor or parishioners by demands of the family; and secondary gains via attention or indulgence of hostility by the pastor or others.

The initiation of collaboration is technically rather simple. The pastor and I talk, preferably before I see the patient. In addition to the facts about the illness, I attempt to get data concerning the nature of the pastor-patient-family relationships, who initiated the process of getting help, and the involvement of other members of the parish. I attempt to evaluate not only the reliability and destructiveness of the patient, but also the referring pastor. I consider this call to be no more than a technical obligation and ordinary courtesy due any responsible referring professional. (The absence of such acknowledgment can be offensive and the slighted and unguided pastor may be provoked into sabotaging or merely not supporting therapy, thus defeating the purpose of the consultation.) With this call, I may offer suggestions to clarify some problem in the relationship, especially if it concerns responsibility, and I attempt to anticipate problems the pastor may have later. Ordinarily, I ask both the patient and pastor about the pastor's attendance at the first consultation; usually this is optional, but if the problem is a complex one, with the pastor's being heavily involved or the family being difficult, I may insist on his being present. I always invite the pastor to call me about anything that may arise that makes him feel uncomfortable or in the need of help, e.g., if the people return to him with complaints, desire additional counseling, or appear to be getting more disturbed. If the pastor is not present at the initial consultation, I always acknowledge the visit by a call to him giving my recommendations, impressions, and possible difficulties that may arise. Usually, once patients start a treatment program and benefit from it, they rarely involve the pastor, and we never hear from each other. Occasionally, I have received information from the pastor in cases in which patients seemed to be doing well that pointed up something about which I had not the slightest awareness, and it was very useful. I have had no reason to regret the involvement of the pastor in the treatment process, and it seems to have met a number of problems existing before I started the practice.

The involvement of the family's pastor when the patient was referred by someone else may be worth a trial if the circumstances are serious enough. However, unless I have worked with the pastor previously, the pastor is inclined to be diffident, and the practice has not been too useful, perhaps because the pastor has not taken the responsibility for the referral or chosen the psychiatrist.

Occasionally, I may refer a patient to a clergyman, as when the patient wishes an opinion about a religious matter connected with his problems. While I do not recommend religious observances or prayers, I have occasionally referred severely socially isolated people who were unable to initiate their own social life to a church for the social experience and help.

The above techniques are, to my mind, merely a realistic recognition that for many people, sick and well, the church represents an important part of their philosophy and social existence. This recognition can be helpful in the psychiatrist's task of intervention in illness. The key figure of the religious institution is the pastor, and his abilities and person can be a valuable ally or otherwise.

REFERENCE

1. Boverman, M., and Adams, J. R. Collaboration of psychiatrist and clergyman: A case report. *Family Process* 3:251, 1964.

Psychiatric Treatment in the Context of the Church

C. F. MIDELFORT

INTRODUCTION

The clergy and mental health professionals come together in their concern for interpersonal relations. Both groups of professionals are giving emphasis to social relations and social institutions. Community psychiatry is looking at the influence of social roles and social institutions on mental well-being—one major institution being the church. Likewise, the church is turning toward its role of responsibility to the lives and well-being of its people, as well as to major social issues, as one of its basic missions [1, 4].

This chapter will focus on some of the social structures, roles, and functions of the church as they influence mental health and illness. Specific illustrations will be given of opportunities for the psychiatrist to work therapeutically, not only with individual church members but also with church institutional roles and structures, in order to achieve health and reintegration of the patient with himself and with his church community.

Although the illness with which the clergy and the mental health professionals are concerned may be seen in different perspectives, the process of illness involves a whole person. Hence, it is natural for the clergy and psychiatrist to come together to treat the spiritual and mental problems that inevitably are present. Since religious

293

groups or communities, large or small, may suffer from rigid structures and illness, the two professions of clergy and psychiatrist should be involved in the treatment. To date, this has largely not materialized. The writer will discuss some groups in which combined therapy has been experienced and indicate where joint effort is urgently needed.

MENTAL HEALTH AND CHURCH ORGANIZATIONS

To begin with, the World Council of Churches is up to the present time untouched by psychiatry. The movement today is shifting emphasis from grace and faith to social action. The needs of nations, of races, of the poor and oppressed demand the concern and action of the Christian churches. There is so little time, and what psychiatry has to offer seems to take so much time. The failure of the church and its people is due in considerable measure to mental and spiritual ills not diagnosed or treated. For example, the paranoid illness that separates East and West has not even been considered from the psychiatric point of view. The obstacles to solving the practical social problems of the world must be reviewed before any imaginative and creative solutions can be found. An intimacy must be developed in which equality is achieved, and a responsibility must be assured that respects real differences. This is the problem of psychotherapy and of "I-Thou" relationships.

The Ecumenical movement consists of different denominations who worship God in each their own traditional manner. This is where the churches stand condemned when the denominations come together to solve some social problem. The social problem is the pretext for common action. Yet little will be accomplished before there is healing of psychological, cultural, social, and spiritual estrangement. This healing comes about when the intimacy of common weakness is discovered and when responsible loyalty to real differences is admitted.

DENOMINATIONAL PROGRAMS

The next involvement of clergy with psychiatrists is at the denominational level. For example, the Episcopal church uses the mental health team to screen its candidates for the priesthood. Each bishop has his own psychiatrist. Each province meets yearly to discuss the mental health of the clergy. At these meetings, bishops and their mental health teams come together to work out practical plans for dealing with such problems as alcoholism or homosexuality among the clergy. The bishop has convocation for his clergy, and the psychiatrist is invited to discuss the relationships of religion and psychotherapy. A major issue confronting the psychiatrist is the fact that church institutional structure may have intrinsic structural elements that are inimical to the health of its members or leaders. Thus, the psychiatrist is faced not only with treating the patient, but also with responding in a helpful and therapeutic manner to the institution that is part of the patient's life.

The joint action of the psychiatrist and the church institution is illustrated in the following case:

A 36-year-old single Episcopalian priest was referred by his bishop, who became concerned when the priest acted as though he were the bishop in suggesting that disciplinary action be taken against a fellow priest for conduct unbefitting a priest. The bishop insisted the priest bring formal charges before the appropriate committee. When the patient could not substantiate his charges before this group, and broke down, the bishop reprimanded the priest, in front of the psychiatrist, for his lack of charity and humility and for acting as if he were the bishop.

The patient was concerned with symbols, all of which seemed to have a sexual meaning. He also thought the bishop and therapist were involved in a plan to change the diocese through group dynamics. This might either save or ruin the diocese.

This illness was related to that of his mother 18 years before. She had thought her husband, a priest, was Joseph and herself Mary and

her son Christ. She had been hospitalized and had received many
electroconvulsive treatments. Now, during her son's illness, she and
her husband came to stay with him and to take part in sessions with
the psychiatrist.

The patient expressed his hostility toward his mother for digging
into the past and toward his father for not having been an adequate
husband. The mother, who also had not previously understood her
own illness, now found things falling into place as she suddenly had
flashes of insight while staying with her son.

The bishop and local parish dismissed the patient from his position and he sought and obtained another position in another state.
His illness represented an excess of fantasy over reality. The
autistic plan to change the diocese and the many sexual fantasies
and symbols were entirely fantasies. Therapy consisted of bringing
the reality of the bishop and of the parents into therapy so that
fantasies could be repressed and the psychosis relieved. It was impossible to modify the sexual picture beyond repressing the fantasies,
because the patient had vowed that he would keep the single state
when he was a boy. At age 12, he had injured his testicles straddling
a fence. Both he and his father had dressed once as women. The
patient had become devoted to a Shrine of Our Lady also in his
adolescence. On several occasions, he had been accused of ruining
male parishioners' spiritual lives by being overly harsh in his treatment of them. His fantasies about men, including his father, his
parishioners, his fellow priests, and the bishop, were negative and
hostile, while his relationships with women were that of defender
and special friend of his mother, the woman supposedly seduced,
the bishop's wife, and the opinion leader of his parish, an elderly
lady.

The problem of this priest shows how the structure of the diocese
was too rigid. The bishop was the rector for the mission church, and
the priest was in a subservient position for years. The fantasies of
this priest grew and expanded until reality was engulfed and relationships became inappropriate. The priest acted as his own bishop,
thereby revolting against the structure. This rebellion threatened
the existence of a fellow priest, the authority of the bishop, and

the welfare of parishioners and parish. Associated with this destructive community relationship was the structure of the priest's family. In the past, the mother's fantasies of being the Virgin Mary, her husband being Joseph, and her son being Christ had so dominated reality that she was unable to distinguish between the cancer of her roommate in the hospital and her own illness. Her fantasies were suppressed by electroconvulsive therapy, but when her son's fantasies dominated his reality years later, her fantasies again came to the fore, and she went through her illness once more. In the family, the father, also a priest, was seen as authoritarian and the mother as an oppressed slave who, with the patient, had to rebel through illness to obtain freedom to be healed or destroyed. Healing took place when the bishop, with his authority, forced the patient to control his fantasies. When the patient wept and kissed the bishop's ring and the bishop reprimanded and relieved him of his parish, there was an intimacy and responsibility that promoted healing. The therapist brought patient, father, and mother together. Mother and son shared an intimacy, she in the flashbacks from her former illness, and he in the sexual symbols that expressed his need for intimacy. She admitted that her life as a mother had been superficial and worldly. The son saw his parents' marriage as lacking in intimacy. He had taken a vow to remain single, and his lack of intimacy had driven him to condemn his fellow priest for being able to be on intimate terms with some of his female parishioners. Equality was found in the weaknesses of mother and son, and responsible reality relationships were preserved by the bishop and father.

HOSPITAL PROGRAMS

The psychiatrist can be of help to the clergy in the Christian medical field of his denomination. The Institute of Human Ecology of the American Lutheran Church is concerned with the hospital care of the whole sick person and his family. The theological, social, cultural, physical, and psychiatric dimensions are all given attention when a person is cared for by them. The nature of hospital structure, of staff relationships with administration, of patients with staff, of hospital with community, all involve the healing ministries of psychiatrist, chaplain, physician, nurse, social worker, family, congregation, and community.

In each group, relationships must be developed in which each person and each representative of the various disciplines heals the other so that they, in turn, may also heal. Acknowledgment of human weakness leads to the equality and intimacy of a full realization of each other's roles and positions. These processes become a healing experience. Practical problems can serve as foci of attention through which the psychiatrist can help the various members of the institution to overcome rigidities and help each other.

SEMINARY PROGRAMS

A psychiatrist who teaches at a seminary has an opportunity to confront the Church with the world and to be confronted by the salvation system of the Church. There seem to be two Christianities, the one that lives in the Church, with its Bible, faith, and salvation, and the other that lives in the world, with its problems. The one finds Christ in the Church, the other in relationships between people that serve and have human needs. Often, an untenable dichotomy is set up. The clergy speaks for the first type of Christianity. It speaks for God. The psychiatrist speaks for man. The clergy controls the animal and spiritual aspects of man. The psychiatrist accepts the animal and spiritual as one. Man is allowed to be animal, but as a responsible animal he may become a Christian. The clergy deplores man's animal nature and says only by faith in Christ can one transcend the animal nature and gain a spiritual nature. There is fakery in the clergy's attitude toward man, and there is a phoniness in the psychiatrist's denial of transcendence. When both can admit their falseness, their weaknesses, their sin of estrangement from one another, an equality will be established that will heal the church and the therapist.

INDIVIDUAL CRISES IN THE CHURCH

Therapeutically, the psychiatrist and the clergy may be seen as having a reciprocal function in treatment: the psychiatrist dealing with the fantasies of the patient, and the clergyman affirming the realities of life. When brought together, these joint forces provide an integrated health-producing experience for the patient [2, 3].

The service of clergy and psychiatrist to a fellow Christian in crisis is shown in the case of the following clergyman.

A 36-year-old single Lutheran pastor had attacks of anxiety with overbreathing, pounding of the heart, blurring of vision, faintness, weakness, and shakiness. His first attack occurred on the way to the dentist. Subsequent spells came on during church service at the point of public confession of sins. His father, a chronic alcoholic, had had little to do with the patient when he was growing up. The mother and maternal grandparents had raised him. Now the senior pastor for whom the patient worked as an assistant found his sermons inadequate and requested that he get a parish of his own.

The "reality" of father and senior pastor who rejected the patient and of the mother and older female Sunday School superintendent who supported the patient produced fantasies of a man who ought to be suppressed. The patient's sex life consisted of masturbation and homosexual relationships. The first anxiety attack, which had occurred on his way to the dentist, was, as he later remembered during therapy, on the day following his being at a dinner with two men, now homosexual partners. One had previously been the patient's homosexual partner.

The patient said he had no guilt over his sexual behavior. The psychiatrist asked the patient if he had ever brought this behavior out in his conversation with the Lord. When he said he had not done this, he was urged to do so. The result was an attack of anxiety in which he felt that he was losing contact with Christ and that his parents were calling him home. He asked to see a pastor of his denomination in order to make a confession and receive Communion. This pastor only heard his confession about masturbation, because the patient was too upset to talk about his homosexuality. The next day he took Communion. The pastor took part in therapeutic sessions during which the present situation with the senior pastor in his church and the future possibilities of having his own parish were discussed.

The patient went home to stay with his parents and became reconciled with his father before the latter died of cirrhosis of the liver. He became interested in the opposite sex and in children and in what it meant to be a parent. After clearing up the remaining responsibilities of his old parish, he took a new position as pastor of a rural church.

This anxiety neurosis can be understood as a suppression of fantasies related to being a senior pastor, and being married and having a family. Fantasy life was restored to him through his prayers, his confession, his Communion, his therapy, and his life with his parents. In keeping with this new fantasy life, reality became more challenging in his accepting a new position and reconciling with his father.

The patient's distorted religion was revealed in the way he kept his salvation religion in church separated from his worldly life of homosexuality and rejection of his alcoholic father. The self-deception gave evidence of its presence in his anxiety attacks on the way to the dentist and during the confessional part of the liturgy. His inauthenticity was apparent to his senior pastor, who felt obliged to check his sermons and to force him out into the world as his own boss. The physicians who treated this illness as exclusively diabetes and nervousness, without getting at the true situation, revealed their own shallow evaluation.

The psychiatrist unearthed the relationship of the anxiety attacks to the homosexuality and to the isolated churchly religion of salvation. Bringing the life of sex into the life of prayer brought the spiritual life of the church out into the world of sex. The clergyman who took part in therapy represented the healing ministry, not only in the confession and communion services, but also in the discussion about the work yet to be done by the patient in his older congregation and in the new parish, where he would be a whole man. The psychiatrist supported the patient as a man reconciled with his alcoholic father and ready to entertain and develop heterosexual fantasies about family life. The patient did heal his relationship with his father and did assume an authentic role as shepherd of a flock.

The anxiety attacks expressed a rebellion against the rigid structure of his home and his church. His father's domination of the family through alcoholism influenced the patient's retreat from the family into his feminine passivity and irresponsible homosexuality. The church's rigidity was seen in the senior pastor's authoritarianism and the patient's ineffectiveness. The therapeutic situation was flexible enough to include psychiatrist and clergy in the same interviews. The radical nature of Christianity was shown in the bringing of the human (sexual) and the spiritual together in relationship through conversation, confession, Communion, and psychotherapy. The two therapists were representatives of the incarnation, in that flesh and blood and transcendental idealism were made one.

The psychiatrist and clergyman may cooperate without taking part in common interviews: the church and the hospital, though in separate buildings, may mutually provide nurture for a person in life, as the following case shows.

A 22-year-old single woman repeatedly cut herself on the arms, using a razor blade. Her father had died an alcoholic, her mother a drug addict. The mother had put her daughter up on a pedestal, protected her from life, but when under the influence of drugs showed her what hell was like. From an early age the patient withdrew from life. To please her mother, she studied piano and got good marks in school. After the death of her parents, she became obsessed with the idea of suicide.

Her Wisconsin Synod Lutheran pastor preached hellfire and hatred of sin and human nature to the degree that she hated herself and wished to die. For a while, she freed herself from this tyranny by becoming an atheist. She joined the Unitarian-Universalist Fellowship, but also began to attend the Episcopal Church. The priest ministered to her, and she sought refuge from her suicidal urges by going to his church or calling him on the phone. He always helped her, and he brought her to the hospital and arranged for her to have psychotherapy.

During therapy she felt a compulsion to hug her friends, the priest, and the psychiatrist. This physical contact brought her back from her withdrawn periods of unreality. Suicide became an impossible way of escaping life, and she proceeded forward to find her humanness and that of others.

The rigidity of her Lutheran church and of her family was apparent in the pastor's hateful authoritarianism and in her parents' use of alcohol and drugs to avoid reality. The reality of humanness, where body, feelings, trust, faith, and commitment are possible, was discovered in the Episcopal Church and in the hospital. The priest and psychiatrist both committed themselves to her, and she gradually broke down the "marble wall" surrounding herself. Openness, sharing, creativity, and equality were experienced. She permitted the therapist to come down from the pedestal, and she came out of the abyss to meet him halfway in honest dialogue. Her guilt, jealousy, and fragmentation decreased as she accepted more sides to her person and to his. The pedestal-abyss structure of home and church was replaced by a real caring, trusting, and accepting.

CONCLUSION

The preceding are examples of crises in life in which psychiatrist and clergy must collaborate. Various levels of involvement, from the largest to the smallest, from groups to individuals, have been presented. They involve spiritual and mental health for the world, the nation, the denomination, the seminary, the diocese, and the individual pastor. The mental health team represented by the psychiatrist has something practical and important to contribute to the welfare of us all. The process of living brings physical, spiritual, and mental health together. The inauthentic in us must be exposed before healing can take place and the practical crises be met.

REFERENCES

1. Lambourne, R. A. *Community, Church, and Healing.* London: Darton, Longman and Todd, 1963.
2. Midelfort, C. F. *The Family in Psychotherapy.* New York: McGraw-Hill, 1957.
3. Midelfort, C. F. Use of members of the family in the treatment of schizophrenia. *Fam. Process* 1:114, 1962.
4. Wilson, M. *The Church Is Healing.* Naperville, Ill.: SCM Books, 1966.

A Contemporary Bibliography on Psychiatry and Religion

The aim of this bibliography is to provide a brief, topical reference guide to the clinician. Thus, the classical literature in the psychology of religion, the classic psychoanalytic studies of religion, and books of a more theological or pastoral nature have been omitted for brevity. Each topic is not covered exhaustively, but rather, representative salient books are listed. In several areas there is still a paucity of sophisticated literature. Emphasis has been placed on works of contemporary relevance that are based on clinical, experimental, or philosophical rigor.

I. PSYCHIATRY AND RELIGION—GENERAL TEXTS

Braceland, F. J., and Stock, M. *Modern Psychiatry: A Handbook for Believers.* New York: Doubleday, 1963.

Gassert, R. G., and Hall, B. H. *Psychiatry and Religious Faith.* New York: Viking Press, 1964.

Knight, J. A. *A Psychiatrist Looks at Religion and Health.* New York: Abingdon, 1964.

Linn, L., and Schwarz, L. W. *Psychiatry and Religious Experience.* New York: Random House, 1958.

Meehl, P. (Ed.). *What, Then, Is Man? A Symposium of Theology, Psychology and Psychiatry.* St. Louis: Concordia, 1958.

Noveck, S. (Ed.). *Judaism and Psychiatry.* New York: Basic Books, 1956.

Psychiatry and religion: Some steps toward mutual understanding and usefulness. *Group Advance. Psychiat.* [*Rep.*] 48, 1960.
The psychic function of religion in mental illness and health. *Group Advance. Psychiat.* [*Rep.*] 67, 1968.
Some considerations of early attempts in cooperation between religion and psychiatry. *Group Advance. Psychiat.* [*Sympos.*] 5, 1958.

II. PSYCHOANALYSIS AND RELIGION

Erikson, E. H. *Young Man Luther.* New York: W. W. Norton, 1958.
Fromm, E. *Psychoanalysis and Religion.* New Haven, Conn.: Yale University Press, 1950.
Meng, H., and Freud, E. L. (Ed.). *Sigmund Freud: Psychoanalysis and Faith. Dialogues with the Reverend Oskar Pfister.* New York: Basic Books, 1963.
Ostow, M., and Scharfstein, B. A. *The Need to Believe: The Psychology of Religion.* New York: International Universities Press, 1954.
Rieff, P. *Freud: The Mind of the Moralist.* New York, Viking, 1959.
Zilboorg, G. *Psychoanalysis and Religion.* New York: Farrar, Straus & Cudahy, 1962.

III. EXISTENTIAL PSYCHOTHERAPY AND RELIGION

Allers, R. *Existentialism and Psychiatry.* Springfield, Ill.: C. C. Thomas, 1961.
Benda, C. *The Image of Love.* New York: Free Press, 1961.
Caruso, I. A. *Existential Psychology: From Analysis to Synthesis.* New York: Herder & Herder, 1964.
Daim, W. *Depth Psychology and Salvation.* New York: F. Ungar, 1963.
Frankl, V. E. *Man's Search for Meaning: An Introduction to Logotherapy.* Boston: Beacon Press, 1962.
Stern, K. *The Third Revolution: A Study of Psychiatry and Religion.* London: Michael Joseph, 1955.

IV. VALUES, MORALITY, AND PSYCHOTHERAPY

Birmingham, W., and Cunneen, J. E. (Eds.). *Cross Currents of Psychiatry and Catholic Morality.* New York: Pantheon Books, 1963.

Erikson, E. H. *Insight and Responsibility.* New York: W. W. Norton, 1964.

Halmos, P. *The Faith of the Counsellors.* New York: Schocken Books, 1966.

Hartmann, H. *Psychoanalysis and Moral Values.* New York: International Universities Press, 1960.

London, P. *The Modes and Morals of Psychotherapy.* New York: Holt, Rinehart & Winston, 1964.

Margolis, J. *Psychotherapy and Morality.* New York: Random House, 1966.

Moral Values in Psychoanalysis. Symposium No. 6. New York: Academy of Religion and Mental Health, 1965.

Rieff, P. *The Triumph of the Therapeutic: Uses of Faith After Freud.* New York: Harper & Row, 1966.

V. PSYCHOPATHOLOGY AND RELIGION

Boisen, A. T. *Out of the Depths.* New York: Harper, 1960.

Frank, J. D. *Persuasion and Healing.* Baltimore: Johns Hopkins Press, 1961.

Festinger, L., Riecken, H. W., and Shachter, S. *When Prophecy Fails.* Minneapolis: University of Minnesota Press, 1956.

Hoffer, E. *The True Believer.* New York: Mentor Books, 1951.

La Barre, W. *They Shall Take Up Serpents. Psychology of the Southern Snake-Handling Cult.* Minneapolis: University of Minnesota Press, 1962.

Oates, W. E. *Religious Factors in Mental Illness.* London: George Allen & Unwin, 1957.

Rokeach, M. *The Three Christs of Ypsilanti.* New York: Knopf, 1964.

Sargant, W. *Battle for the Mind.* New York: Doubleday, 1957.

VI. COMMUNITY MENTAL HEALTH AND RELIGION

Clinebell, H. J., Jr. *Mental Health Through Christian Community.* Nashville: Abingdon, 1964.

Dittes, J. E. *The Church in the Way.* New York: Scribner's, 1967.
Hoffman, H. (Ed.). *The Ministry and Mental Health.* New York: Association Press, 1960.
Johnson, F. E. (Ed.). *Religion and Social Work.* New York: Harper, 1956.
Klausner, S. Z. *Psychiatry and Religion: A Sociological Study of the New Alliance of Ministers and Psychiatrists.* New York: Free Press, 1964.
McCann, R. V. *The Churches and Mental Health.* New York: Basic Books, 1962.
Maves, P. B. (Ed.). *The Church and Mental Health.* New York: Scribner's, 1953.
Oglesby, W. B. *Referral in Pastoral Counseling.* Englewood, N.J.: Prentice-Hall, 1968.
Palmer, C. E. *Religion and Rehabilitation.* Springfield, Ill.: C. C. Thomas, 1968.
Westberg, G. E., and Draper, E. *Community Psychiatry and the Clergyman.* Springfield, Ill.: C. C. Thomas, 1966.

VII. MENTAL HEALTH AND RELIGIOUS VOCATIONS

Bowers, M. *Conflicts of the Clergy.* New York: T. Nelson, 1963.
Denton, W. *The Role of the Minister's Wife.* Philadelphia: Westminster, 1962.
Douglas, W. *Ministers' Wives.* New York: Harper & Row, 1965.
Evoy, J. J., and Christoph, V. F. *Personality Development in the Religious Life.* New York: Sheed & Ward, 1963.
Kennedy, E. C., and D'Arcy, P. F. *The Genius of the Apostolate: Personal Growth in the Candidate, the Seminarian, and the Priest.* New York: Sheed & Ward, 1965.
Oates, W. E. *The Minister's Own Mental Health.* Great Neck, N.Y.: Channel Press, 1961.
Vaughn, R. P. *Mental Illness and the Religious Life.* Milwaukee: Bruce, 1962.

VIII. ASSESSMENT OF RELIGIOUS CANDIDATES

Arnold, M. B. (Ed.). *Screening Candidates for the Priesthood and Religious Life.* Chicago: Loyola University Press, 1962.
Coville, W. J. (Ed.). *Assessment of Candidates for the Religious*

Life. Washington, D.C.: Center for Applied Research Apostolate, 1968.

IX. PSYCHOLOGY OF RELIGION

Allport, G. W. *The Individual and His Religion.* New York: Macmillan, 1962.

Clark, W. H. *The Psychology of Religion.* New York: Macmillan, 1958.

Havens, J. (Ed.). *Psychology and Religion: A Contemporary Dialogue.* Princeton, N.J.: D. Van Nostrand, 1968.

Johnson, P. E. *The Psychology of Religion.* Nashville: Abingdon, 1958.

Pruyser, P. *A Dynamic Psychology of Religion.* New York: Harper & Row, 1968.

Spinks, G. S. *Psychology and Religion: An Introduction to Contemporary Views.* Boston: Beacon Press, 1965.

Strunk, O., Jr. (Ed.). *Readings in the Psychology of Religion.* Nashville: Abingdon, 1959.

X. SOCIAL PSYCHOLOGY OF RELIGION

Argyle, M. *Religious Behavior.* Glencoe, Ill.: Free Press, 1958.

Glock, C. Y., and Stark, R. *Religion and Society in Tension.* Chicago: Rand McNally, 1965.

Hopkins, P. *The Social Psychology of Religious Experience.* New York: Paine-Whitman, 1963.

Lenski, G. *The Religious Factor.* New York: Doubleday, 1961.

Rokeach, M. *Beliefs, Values, and Attitudes.* San Francisco: Jossey-Bass, 1968.

Whiteley, O. R. *Religious Behavior: Where Sociology and Religion Meet.* Englewood Cliffs, N.J.: Prentice-Hall, 1964.

XI. CULTURAL PSYCHIATRY AND RELIGION

Boisen, A. T. *Religion in Crisis and Custom: A Sociological and Psychological Study.* New York: Harper, 1955.

Kiev, A. (Ed.). *Magic, Faith, and Healing. Studies in Primitive Psychiatry Today.* New York: Free Press, 1964.

Kiev, A. *Curanderismo: Mexican-American Folk Psychiatry.* New York: Free Press, 1968.
Religion, Culture, and Mental Health. Symposium No. 3. New York: Academy of Religion and Mental Health, 1961.
Soddy, K. (Ed.). *Identity, Mental Health and Value Systems.* Chicago: Quadrangle Books, 1961.
Wallace, A. F. C. *Religion: An Anthropological View.* New York: Random House, 1966.

XII. PERSONALITY DEVELOPMENT AND RELIGION

Godin, A. (Ed.). *Child and Adult Before God.* Chicago: Loyola University Press, 1965.
Godin, A. (Ed.). *From Religious Experience to a Religious Attitude.* Chicago: Loyola University Press, 1965.
Goldman, R. *Religious Thinking from Childhood to Adolescence.* London: Humanities Press, 1966.
Lewis, E. *Children and Their Religion.* New York: Sheed & Ward, 1962.
Loomis, E. A., Jr. *The Self in Pilgrimage.* New York: Harper, 1960.
Religion in the Developing Personality. Symposium No. 2. New York: Academy of Religion and Mental Health, 1960.
Rosen, B. C. *Adolescence and Religion.* Cambridge: Schenkman, 1965.
Stewart, C. W. *Adolescent Religion.* New York: Abingdon, 1967.

XIII. PERSONALITY THEORY AND RELIGION

Doniger, S. (Ed.). *The Nature of Man in Theological and Psychological Perspective.* New York: Harper, 1962.
Hiltner, S., and Menninger, K. (Eds.). *Constructive Aspects of Anxiety.* Nashville: Abingdon, 1963.
Lapsley, J. N. *The Concept of Willing.* New York: Abingdon, 1967.
McKenzie, J. G. *Guilt: Its Meaning and Significance.* New York: Abingdon, 1962.
Oates, W. E. *Religious Dimensions of Personality.* New York: Association Press, 1957.

Oraison, M. (Ed.). *A Symposium.* New York: Macmillan, 1962.
Roberts, D. *Psychotherapy and a Christian View of Man.* New York: Scribner's, 1950.
Royce, J. E. *Man and Meaning* (revised). New York: McGraw-Hill, 1969.
Van Kaam, A. L. *Religion and Personality.* Englewood Cliffs, N.J.: Prentice-Hall, 1964.

XIV. PSYCHOLOGY OF RELIGIOUS EXPERIENCES

Brantl, G. (Ed.). *The Religious Experience* (2 vols.). New York: G. Braziller, 1964.
de Sanctis, S. *Religious Conversion.* London: Kegan, Paul, Trench, Trubner, 1927.
Goodenough, E. R. *The Psychology of Religious Experiences.* New York: Basic Books, 1965.
Gordon, A. I. *The Nature of Conversion.* Boston: Beacon Press, 1967.
Laski, M. *Ecstasy: A Study of Some Religious and Secular Experiences.* Bloomington, Ind.: Indiana University Press, 1961.
Maslow, A. H. *Religions, Values, and Peak-Experiences.* Columbus, Ohio: Ohio State University Press, 1964.
Stace, W. T. *Mysticism and Philosophy.* New York: Lippincott, 1960.
Underhill, E. *Mysticism: A Study of the Nature and Development of Man's Spiritual Consciousness.* New York: Meridian Books, 1955.

XV. THEOLOGY AND PSYCHOTHERAPY

Browning, D. S. *Atonement and Psychotherapy.* Philadelphia: Westminster, 1966.
Hulme, W. E. *Counseling and Theology.* Philadelphia: Muhlenberg, 1956.
Oden, T. C. *Contemporary Theology and Psychotherapy.* Philadelphia: Westminster, 1967.
Outler, A. C. *Psychotherapy and the Christian Message.* New York: Harper, 1954.

XVI. PASTORAL CARE AND COUNSELING

Clinebell, H. J., Jr. *Basic Types of Pastoral Counseling.* Nashville: Abingdon, 1966.

Draper, E. *Psychiatry and Pastoral Care.* Englewood Cliffs, N.J.: Prentice-Hall, 1965.

Hiltner, S. *Preface to Pastoral Theology.* New York: Abingdon, 1958.

McNeill, J. T. *The History of the Cure of Souls.* New York: Harper, 1951.

Wise, C. A. *The Meaning of Pastoral Care.* New York: Harper & Row, 1966.

XVII. RESEARCH STUDIES

Cook, S. W. (Ed.). *Research Plans in the Fields of Religion, Values and Morality.* New York: Religious Education Association, 1962.

Cook, S. W. (Ed.). *Review of Recent Research Bearing on Religious and Character Formation.* New York: Religious Education Association, 1962.

Hathorne, B. C. *Research Monograph: A Critical Analysis of Protestant Church Counseling Centers.* Washington, D.C.: General Board of Christian Social Concerns, Methodist Church, 1964.

Hiltner, S., and Colston, H. G. *The Context of Pastoral Counseling.* New York: Abingdon, 1961.

Research in Religion and Health. Symposium No. 5. New York: Academy of Religion and Mental Health, 1961.

Rokeach, M. *The Open and Closed Mind.* New York: Basic Books, 1960.

XVIII. BIBLIOGRAPHIES

Albert, E. M., and Kluckhohn, C. *A Selected Bibliography on Values, Ethics, and Esthetics.* Glencoe, Ill.: Free Press, 1959.

Berkowitz, J. J., and Johnson, J. E. *Social Scientific Studies of Religion: A Bibliography.* Pittsburgh: University of Pittsburgh Press, 1967.

Bibliography on Religion and Mental Health: 1960-1964. Public Health Service Publication No. 1599. Washington, D.C.: U.S. Government Printing Office, 1967.

Meissner, W. W. *Annotated Bibliography in Religion and Psychology.* New York: Academy of Religion and Mental Health, 1961.

Menges, R. J., and Dittes, J. E. *Psychological Studies of Clergymen: Abstracts of Research.* New York: T. Nelson, 1965.

Index

315